THE
MIRACLE PILL

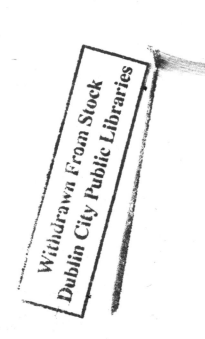

THE MIRACLE PILL

Why a Sedentary World is Getting it All Wrong

PETER WALKER

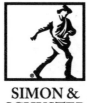

SIMON &
SCHUSTER

London · New York · Sydney · Toronto · New Delhi

First published in Great Britain by Simon & Schuster UK Ltd, 2021

Copyright © Peter Walker, 2021

The right of Peter Walker to be identified as the author of this work has been
asserted in accordance with the Copyright, Designs and Patents Act, 1988.

1 3 5 7 9 10 8 6 4 2

Simon & Schuster UK Ltd
1st Floor
222 Gray's Inn Road
London WC1X 8HB

www.simonandschuster.co.uk
www.simonandschuster.com.au
www.simonandschuster.co.in

Simon & Schuster Australia, Sydney
Simon & Schuster India, New Delhi

The author and publishers have made all reasonable efforts to contact
copyright-holders for permission, and apologise for any omissions or errors in the form
of credits given. Corrections may be made to future printings.

A CIP catalogue record for this book
is available from the British Library.

Hardback ISBN: 978-1-4711-9252-4
Trade Paperback ISBN: 978-1-4711-9253-1
eBook ISBN: 978-1-4711-9254-8

Typeset in Stone Serif by M Rules
Printed in the UK by CPI Group (UK) Ltd, Croydon, CR0 4YY

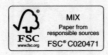

For Ralph

Contents

INTRODUCTION

A World Transformed

Cast your mind back across the past few weeks, and think about how many times you really used your body as part of everyday life. I'm not talking about formal exercise. This isn't a listless jog around the local park, or a spin class squeezed between work chores and family duties, motivated in part by guilt at the thought of the monthly gym fee. I mean using your body in a way that was at least a bit strenuous, and would also be more or less comprehensible to, say, someone from Edwardian times. Perhaps striding across town to an engagement, or digging a garden. Maybe cycling up a hill, not dressed in Lycra and as a penance for too much cake, but to fetch something from a shop. If, right now, you're struggling to immediately recall anything on these lines, you are by no means alone.

It is fair to say that there is a modern crisis when it comes to physical movement. In the UK, well over three in ten of the adult population lead lives so inactive that their long-term health could be harmed.[1] That's more than 20 million people. An alarming 80 per cent of British children exert themselves so little that they risk growing up with weakened bones, poorly developed cardiovascular systems, and bodies more likely to suffer from chronic illness as they age.[2] You can find similar statistics for more or less any other economically developed country in the world, and increasingly for many poorer ones. Possibly the most exhaustive global study, which combined data from 122 nations, found that nearly a third of all adults, and four fifths of adolescents, currently move insufficiently in their lives.[3]

What has happened? The short answer is that everyday physical activity more or less disappeared from the world. Regular, informal, unplanned exertion, an integral part of virtually every human life since the first *Homo sapiens* hunted and foraged, was designed out of existence, and with astonishing rapidity. This process began in the nineteenth century, with mass industrialisation and urbanisation, but has accelerated almost beyond measure in recent decades. It has involved everything from the decline of physical work in favour of desk-based jobs, to homes filled with activity-saving devices, where even mini-exertions like walking to the cinema or a restaurant are being gradually replaced by streamed films and the rise of app-summoned takeaways. The same has happened to our external environment, where the routine effort of walking and cycling has been supplanted by ubiquitous car journeys, many of them carrying one person for a laughably short distance.

This transformation has been so rapid as to put much of it within living memory. Even in the economically booming UK of the mid-to-late 1950s, barely half of households owned a vacuum cleaner,[4] while only a quarter possessed a washing machine, and even many of those who had the latter still used a mangle to dry their clothes.[5] Millions of older Britons can thus still recall a human-powered domestic regime of rug beating and hand-washed clothes almost unaltered from the nineteenth century. In the same post-war Britain, around 70 per cent of jobs involved manual labour, as against fewer than a third currently.[6] In 1950, around 25 per cent of all trips were still made by bicycle.[7] These days that figure is somewhere near 1 per cent,[8] with cycling levels so low it is difficult to be more precise. About a quarter of all journeys of less than two miles, the sort of distance you could cycle fairly sedately in ten or fifteen minutes, are done by car.[9]

Some of the statistics around inactivity can be genuinely jaw-dropping. In a recent study, Public Health England, the government body charged with improving the nation's wellbeing, asked people how much cumulative time *in an average month* they spent walking briskly. Not jogging, or even a gentle trot, just a slightly increased walking pace. The answer from 44 per cent was, 'Less than ten minutes' – that is, pretty much not at all.[10] Another example comes in the Annual Travel Survey, an examination by the UK's Department for Transport into the various methods people used to get around over the previous twelve months. The most recent edition, from 2018, asked how many times during the previous year the 15,000-plus panel had walked continuously for twenty minutes or longer. This meant walking at any speed, not even briskly. A whole 18 per cent ticked the box saying, 'Less than once a year'. Again – pretty much never.[11]

There is another element to this physical revolution. The void created by the disappearance of routine movement has, in part, been filled with the notion of exercise, something separate from your everyday life, increasingly commercialised, even fetishised, and thus far from universal. Over recent decades the fitness industry has boomed worldwide, barely making a dent in overall activity levels but allowing governments to focus on the idea of sport as a substitute.

This is not meant as a condemnation of gym-going or any other type of formal sport. They bring joy and fulfilment to millions, not to mention enormous health benefits. Your body doesn't care how you exert yourself. The only problem is that not enough people do it. In the UK, more than half the adult population never take part in any sport, ever.[12] But the attention devoted to exercise rather than everyday movement has helped shift the public narrative towards one based on oversimplified notions of personal responsibility, as if declining activity levels were caused by nothing more than a mass outbreak of laziness.

This not only entirely misses the point, but provides an excuse for politicians not to treat inactivity with the complete seriousness it merits. And make no mistake: this is one of the more momentous changes in recent human existence. To get a sense of the scale, consider the findings of what is almost certainly the most thorough academic attempt to total up the number of global deaths each year connected to inactive living. The figure reached was 5.3 million. That's about the population of Norway, dying earlier than they should.[13] It is more than are killed in wars,[14] and in many countries more than by tobacco.[15] A tally by UK health officials estimates the national death toll due to inactive living at around 100,000 a year.[16] By the same gauge of measurement, that's a small city, something of the size of Worcester. It's more than 270 people a day – almost 60 per day more than tobacco.

But the impact goes far beyond mortality statistics and the associated human tragedy they contain. With countless millions of people acquiring lifestyle-related illnesses like type 2 diabetes at ever-earlier ages, and living for many more decades with a series of chronic, debilitating conditions, most experts agree that, if left unchecked, inactivity is on course to make health services fundamentally unviable. This is very much a question of when, not if.

A World Transformed

In the six-plus decades since a pioneering British researcher first demonstrated the link between a lack of movement in people's everyday lives and chronic illness, knowledge about the sheer range of perils it can cause has multiplied. Many thousands of subsequent studies have clearly established that inactive living, if maintained over years and decades, brings an increased likelihood of not just type 2 diabetes and other metabolic disorders, but heart disease, high blood pressure and strokes, several forms of cancer, poor lung function, as well as depression and anxiety, diminished cognitive function, poorer sleep and, in later life, Alzheimer's and other sorts of dementia. Not to mention the big ones: increased chances of early death, or, if you do survive into retirement, a reduced chance of being able to live healthily and independently.

Inactive living is also a key factor in the connected but distinct global health catastrophe of excess weight and obesity. Finally, there is the parallel blight of ailments caused by people sitting down too long, which is also heavily linked to type 2 diabetes and cardiovascular disease.

Dr Adrian Davies is a British academic who has spent more than thirty years researching ways to keep people moving. He is clear about where we find ourselves: 'In terms of rigour in science and public health we are at that stage where we absolutely know that *Homo sapiens* were designed, as hunter-gatherers, to be routinely physically active, chasing antelopes across the prairie or whatever it was. And while we have not been able to change our biological destiny, we have changed the built environment. So instead of hunting an antelope we get in the car and drive to Sainsbury's.'[17]

This book is the story of how routine activity disappeared, and the many consequences it brought. There are several things this book is not. It is not an argument for simply turning back the clock. No one wants a return to mass, repetitive manual labour. And beyond a handful of hair-shirted survivalist types, few would suggest having to carry in piles of wood from a shed every day for heating and cooking. Similarly, domestic appliances like the washing machine and vacuum cleaner have liberated millions of people – almost universally women – from hours of daily drudgery. This is, instead, about finding new ways to put physical effort into modern lives.

Nor is this intended as a handbook for better health, or a detailed policy manifesto. There are plenty of those already available. Consider it more a guide through this often unnoticed phenomenon and its many consequences, which are hiding in plain sight in virtually every country across the world. But along the way, I hope to point out at least some of the ways through which you might integrate more movement into your routine, and explain the near-magical benefits that can follow. As such, each chapter ends with an idea about how to perhaps integrate more movement into your life. But this is meant just as something to think about, not an instruction, let alone a programme, or a regime.

Because this book is also a story of hope. Even in an environment designed against human-powered motion, change can be easier than you think. It is still possible to experience movement and exertion as a regular part of your life, not just a chore, a penance. Again, this is not to demean sport. But it is just not the same thing. When you make something routine, normal, even forgettable, you no longer need to carve time out of your day to do it, or feel guilty when you don't. Instead it embeds, becomes permanent. When this happens it feels almost as if you have been let in on a secret.

The consequences that follow for your wellbeing can be astounding. The decades of research into the dangers of inactivity have seen a parallel growth in knowledge about the seemingly endless ways that, once you start moving again, the health odds begin to stack once more in your favour, and almost instantly. With scientists better able to electronically monitor the subtleties and variations of movement and exertion, it has become apparent that even pretty moderate, everyday efforts can bring significant results. The more information emerges, the steeper the dose–response curve seems to be. Almost anything, it seems, is better than nothing.

I will give just one example, which focuses on that most everyday of physical pursuits, cycling for transport. Researchers in Denmark tracked around 30,000 randomly selected people of all ages over about fifteen years. The study found that even after adjusting for other demographic, social and lifestyle factors, including leisure-time exercise, people who cycled to and from work – the average commute was only about fifteen minutes each way – were 40 per cent less likely to have died over the study period than those who did not, from any cause.[18]

Forty per cent. It is this sort of statistic which helps you understand why some experts can go a bit misty-eyed when they talk about activity. It's also why so many of them compare everyday movement to the miracle-giving pill of this book's title.

In the public health world the idea of activity-as-a-wonder-medicine is so common as to be considered something of a cliché, but it's still the most resonant parallel I can find. Imagine if you were a medical researcher and you discovered a drug which would improve people's health outcomes on the scale of cycle commuting. A Nobel Prize would be more or less guaranteed, as would a knighthood or damehood. In fact, the renown would be so great you'd have a decent chance of ending up with your face on a banknote within your lifetime. And yet this marvel is already here.

Escape from inactivity

There is a final element in introducing this story: why is it me telling it? I'm not a scientist, let alone an epidemiologist, the researchers who investigate population-wide health outcomes. I'm a journalist. I cover British politics, based in the Houses of Parliament.

There are two main reasons for my near-obsessive interest in the subject. One is that my day job involves contact with a lot of politicians, civil servants and other officials, trying to understand why they make certain decisions rather than others. And it's fair to say that when it comes to public health, something odd is going on. If I have the chance to turn a conversation with one of these people to physical inactivity, more or less all of them agree that, yes, it is a hugely significant problem and more should be done. And yet more or less nothing is done. Even though its consequences have been well known for decades, inactivity is what you might call a normalised catastrophe. Governments rarely pass laws, or hold urgent press conferences to pledge action, instead focusing on generally ineffective public information campaigns.

Until now, perhaps. By coincidence, this book is being written while the UK and many other countries are in lockdown due to the coronavirus pandemic. And here, as the world has seen, a swift and coherent response to health emergencies is very much politically feasible. Ministers have not hesitated to close whole sections of their national economies and severely restrict individual freedoms to save lives. For the most part, at time of writing, the public have supported these actions. Interventionist health policies are no longer exceptional. And if voters can accept their government effectively locking them in their homes for two months to save lives, perhaps far less intrusive measures to create more everyday activity, for the same reason, are less likely to attract the traditional opposing cry of, 'Nanny state!'

There has also already been material change. As the lockdown has been relaxed, governments are urging those returning to work to walk or cycle, so as to avoid either packing into public transport or jamming the streets with cars. Emergency cycle lanes are springing up in cities around the world. And as we will see later, active travel is one of the very best ways to ensure movement is part of your routine.

So are we entering a new era of government action to banish inactivity, even indirectly? It will be years before we truly know. But a lot of entrenched attitudes will need to shift. Currently, far too much official thinking on the subject remains based around misplaced assumptions. One is that motivation is the missing element in our crisis of immobility, rather than a world redesigned to discourage movement. Another is that if people are inactive then the consequences are theirs alone. This is an issue which not only blights so many individual health outcomes, but on a national level risks bringing down the entire NHS, not to mention the care system for older people. Some crises are just too big to be left to notions of personal responsibility.

But at the same time, it's worth noting that coronavirus has, undeniably, seen a lot of people think consciously, perhaps for the first time in years, about their individual relationships with physical activity. At the peak of the lockdown in the UK, government guidelines permitted an hour of outdoor movement or activity a day – as one public health expert told me, probably the first time ministers had mandated exercise to the nation since the Second World War. Parks started to half-resemble some sort of idealised Victorian sanatorium, full of joggers, brisk walkers, people skipping or lifting weights.

Inside people's homes, hundreds of thousands of families

launched into unfamiliar sequences of star jumps, stomach crunches and press-ups to the on-screen instruction of Joe Wicks, the fitness guru who launched a parallel career as the nation's de facto PE teacher. In a curious inversion, for some Britons, being instructed to shut themselves in their homes for twenty-three hours a day meant they were actually more active than usual.

Even in normal times, people's relationship with activity is never straightforward, and is greatly shaped by their background, and the lives they lead. This takes us to the other reason for my passion about this subject: it is what you could call biographical. The fact that, as an adult, I am regularly active, with all the benefits this brings, came about because of circumstances which were almost accidental but became something for which I am intensely, permanently grateful. It's not an exaggeration to say that everyday movement transformed my life.

A public health expert might argue, with legitimacy, that coming from the relative privilege of a middle-class family, the statistics favoured me in terms of long-term activity and fitness. But my circumstances were not typical, and there was a period in my young adulthood where a gradual drift towards an increasingly immobile life seemed entirely realistic.

As a child, my health was blighted by asthma which developed extremely early, after a near-fatal episode of pneumonia when I was two, and was soon diagnosed as severe. The condition is part hereditary, part environmental, and I had it coming at me from both sides. My father and one of my maternal uncles had been badly asthmatic as children, while my mother smoked prodigiously both during her pregnancy with me and throughout my infancy, damaging my nascent lungs.

I don't want to portray myself as some sort of tubercular Victorian urchin. Apart from intermittent bouts of wheezing

I was an active if alarmingly skinny child, with a passionate interest in playing football, despite my fairly evident lack of talent. But my asthma was serious enough for doctors to try me out on an array of emerging medicines during regular trips to hospital outpatient departments. Things changed when I became a teenager. As can happen with the condition, my asthma improved in daily life but condensed into rare and terrifying episodes of severe wheezing, several of which ended in emergency admissions to hospital. Around 1,400 people a year in the UK currently die because of asthma,[19] and under slightly different circumstances I could easily have been one of them.

As is also common, the condition improved considerably into adulthood, but by then I had pretty much given up all activity except walking. This was partly due to my age – there are reams of statistics showing how childhood movement diminishes into adolescence and onwards – but, more importantly, I had lost faith in my body. Throughout university I was keenly aware of how unprepossessing a physical specimen I presented, ghostly pale and so un-muscular that the idea of wearing shorts, even a short-sleeved T-shirt, filled me with unease. I was also extremely conscious that if I did try anything connected to sport, I found the exertion increasingly difficult. I just wasn't really sure what to do about any of it. Having graduated with no idea what I wanted to pursue as a career, I took up a dull if spectacularly secure job as a university administrator, spending all day at a desk. My path seemed set.

What changed was that I embraced that most basic and inescapable type of everyday activity: a manual job. More specifically, I became a bike courier, or messenger, spending all day pedalling urgent documents around London. Looking back, the reasons behind what appeared a pretty rash career move are still not entirely clear, especially given I'd not regularly ridden a bike since I was about twelve, and there was no set wage – you were paid entirely according to how many deliveries you made. I'd even decided to make the move to an outdoor job in autumn.

In retrospect the decision, which left my office colleagues politely baffled, was motivated as much by boredom as anything else. The university job involved a set series of tasks to complete over the course of a year, and without expending too much effort I'd managed to get them done about two months ahead of schedule, meaning I spent weeks with literally nothing to do. I also harboured vague, if unformed, notions of wanting to become fit, and this seemed one route to making such an outcome inescapable. Most trivially, I perhaps just thought bike couriers looked pretty cool, and as with many young men this was a quantity I both lacked and cherished.

Either way, the deed was done, and requirements as basic as my ability to buy food and pay the rent were suddenly dependent on those same scrawny legs being able to pedal me sufficient distances at a reasonable speed. The initial weeks were pretty terrible – I can remember almost bursting into tears when I saw how small my first wage packet was – but as I learned the trade the money became respectable, then even good.

I also got used to the exertion. Mine was a pretty drastic introduction to everyday movement, going immediately from almost nothing to a job where I would regularly cycle fifty or sixty miles a day, five days a week. But I was twenty-two when I started, an age when even such an untested body as mine tends to be hugely adaptable. First I developed a bit more speed on the bike, then stamina. After a while, in a turn of events that left me as surprised as anyone, my legs developed muscles.

Finally, for perhaps the first time in my life, I acquired that sort of virtuous glow only really seen among the young and physically fit. While I'd be lying to say I didn't enjoy this new look, especially when people I hadn't seen for some time pointed it out, it was the mental transformation that was more significant. It took perhaps six months for me to realise that, without even really noticing it, I had shed my unspoken assumption of physical frailty. In contrast, I suddenly felt I could do anything. That feeling, in varying forms, has never really left me, nor has the lingering sense of wonder and pleasure that comes with it.

It goes without saying that mine is a slightly extreme example. As we will see in the next chapter, most official guidance suggests you aim for a minimum of half an hour a day of moderate activity, while academics will tell you that even as little as ten minutes can do a lot of good. In the context of physical exertion being a miracle pill for human health and wellbeing, by cycling 250-plus miles a week, every week, I self-administered a mega-dose.

Since that sudden career change, which ended up lasting about three years, I've always remained active to greater or lesser degrees. I'm now middle-aged, with a family and a job which is both largely desk-bound and currently, amid the most chaotic political period in recent UK history, pretty frantic. I still cycle to and from work – or I do outside of lockdown – but that was often the most exertion I managed in a day. Researching and writing the book prompted me to look again at this part of my life, as did the restrictions of coronavirus, where my usual routine of bike commuting was halted. In particular, I was curious about whether my now more distinctly modest regime had kept me as physically impregnable as I had perhaps assumed.

I thus submitted myself as a sort of research guinea pig, festooned with electronic gadgets that tracked my movement, the time I spent sitting down, my heart rate, calories burned. I also underwent a series of tests of my fitness and general physical health. We'll hear more about all this in later chapters, but without wishing to spoil the suspense, the data and examinations provided a more mixed picture than even I had expected. Yes, I remained significantly fitter than average. But in a few respects, not least the amount I sit down every day and the subsequent impact on my bodily composition, it seemed I had become a bit complacent. So make no mistake: for me this is very personal.

1

The Long Decline of Everyday Movement

Given this is the story of how our lives have changed so dramatically with the disappearance of everyday physical activity, it's probably best to start at the beginning. And that might be slightly longer ago than you expected. About 12,000 years, in fact.

It was around this time that some of our Neolithic ancestors in what is now the Middle East gave up their hunter-gatherer lifestyle and, over numerous generations, began instead to cultivate crops, domesticate animals and form permanent settlements. This is, of course, not particularly long ago by the standards of human history – *Homo sapiens* had emerged anything up to 300,000 years earlier – but what is now known as the First Agricultural Revolution, or Agrarian Revolution, was the beginning of a settled, more densely populated life, helping bring about the development of new tools, then the specialisation of labour. In other words, the building blocks for modern civilisation.

Any 21st-century human suddenly catapulted to one of these first villages would find life there hugely gruelling and overwhelmingly physical. But it was still more sedate than the hunter-gatherer existence, free of the endless miles of walking required to forage and hunt for prey. And so, over the centuries, something began to happen to these early, home-dwelling humans: their bodies changed.

It has long been known that modern humans have considerably less dense bones than similar-sized primates, something often linked to our distinctive upright walking stance. But a fascinating 2014 study by US and British academics found that bones from humans who lived in hunter-gatherer communities in North America around 7,000 years ago (the agricultural revolutions did not happen everywhere simultaneously) were as strong and dense as those now seen in orangutans. In contrast, bones examined from farmers who lived 700 years ago were 20 per cent lighter. The researchers concluded that this 'gracility' of the more modern skeleton, a rather lovely technical term meaning 'slenderness', was not caused by a changing diet, or by different body sizes as humans evolved, but simply because of reduced physical exertion.[1]

Such change has very modern consequences. Human bone density is significantly affected by how active someone is, particularly during childhood and adolescence, with weight-bearing movements like running and jumping key to this development. Bone density usually peaks in early adulthood and then declines as we age, particularly with women, and all the more so through long-term inactivity. Loss of bone density increases the risk of fractures or the debilitating condition of osteoporosis, another evocative technical term which literally means 'porous bones'. The health impacts are enormous. Studies have shown that among older people who suffer an osteoporosis-related hip injury, up to 20 per cent die in the first year, and two thirds never regain the same level of mobility.[2]

There is some important context to be added: in activity terms, these farmers clearly had much more in common with hunter-gatherers than with today's humans, so any bodily changes were relative. Another study examined bone mass in women from other early agricultural communities, this time in central Europe. It found that while the bones in their legs were generally comparable to those of modern women, with their arms it was a very different story. The humerus, or upper arm bone, showed rigidity and indications of strength comparable or even greater than that of modern-day elite female rowers. These women clearly carried or hoisted sizeable loads on a more or less daily basis, and they had the bone density to prove it.[3]

Gathering a more detailed picture of our ancestors' physical lives is, understandably, not easy, short of using a time machine to attach an activity tracker to a prehistoric farmer's leg. One creative part-answer has come from studying people whose lifestyles have at least something in common with those from the past. A fascinating project saw academics examine activity patterns in a community of Amish people in Ontario, Canada. The Amish are a Protestant group that originated in Switzerland but came to North America in the eighteenth century. As well as following a creed of non-violence, they pursue traditional values to the extent of rejecting all modern technology, meaning that – as regularly portrayed in films and television – their methods for everything from agriculture to travel involve nothing more high-tech than horses and hand-tools.

Luckily for researchers, Amish rules do not completely bar them from using modern inventions, just owning them. That meant the ninety-eight Amish men and women who took part were able to spend a week with an electronic step counter attached to the waistband of their trousers or to an apron – one slight complicating factor was that the Amish are forbidden to wear belts.

When the results arrived, they were striking. Separate surveys have calculated that the average Canadian adult walks just over 4,800 steps per day. In contrast, the Amish men averaged almost 18,500. Even the community's women, who traditionally spend most of their time in domestic and child-rearing activities rather than farming, managed well over 14,000 steps.

The highest individual one-day total was 51,514 steps, more than 20 miles, recorded by an Amish man who was harrowing farmland, the process of smoothing and breaking up soil, while walking behind a team of five Belgian horses. The best for a woman was the 41,176 steps achieved by a farmer's wife who rose at 3:30am to assist with the agricultural chores before beginning her own domestic duties. In such a world the idea of 'exercise' seems redundant. Of the men and women studied, only two – both men – listed leisure activities in the accompanying activity questionnaire, mentioning fishing.[4]

It is a very long time since Amish-style levels of exertion were the norm in places like the UK, a factor of both mechanisation and a shift away from rural life. Britain experienced a particularly early exodus of agricultural populations to factory jobs in towns and cities, with the country's rate of urbanisation soaring from below 50 per cent in 1840 to nearly 80 per cent by the end of that century.[5] But even decades after that, up to the post-war era of the 1950s, although for many people the repetitive physical grind of manual factory labour had been replaced by sedentary work, other aspects of life remained significantly more active than we experience now.

How do we know this for certain? One innovative experiment saw a group of volunteers fitted with sensors to measure how much energy they expended, before being set to work carrying out a series of identical household and transport activities in two different ways. They washed a selection of dishes in a sink, and then loaded the same number into a dishwasher. Dirty clothes were laundered by hand, then re-dirtied and put in a washing machine. An imaginary 0.8-mile commute was done on a treadmill to simulate walking, and then by car. Finally, our long-suffering test subjects ascended and descended a series of floors using the stairs, before doing so in a lift.

The results showed that hand-washing dishes and clothes was, as you would expect, more strenuous than the automated versions, by 40 per cent and 55 per cent respectively. But much greater differences came when the whole body was in motion. The simulated walking commute and the stair climbing were both more than three times as strenuous as letting machinery do the work. Factoring in how often people tend to perform all these tasks on average, the researchers calculated that these modern conveniences meant people now expend 111 fewer calories* per day on average.[6]

This might not seem much, given the recommended daily intake is 2,500 calories for men and 2,000 for women.[7] But as the research paper pointed out, dropping your energy expenditure by 111 calories a day without a parallel reduction in food intake brings an average weight gain of more than 4kg a year, which is a relatively rapid path towards obesity.

Steven Blair is emeritus professor at the Arnold School of Public Health at South Carolina University. He is one of the world's leading experts on how everyday movement has

---

* What is generally called a calorie is officially a 'kilocalorie', which is the amount of energy needed to raise the temperature of a litre of water by one degree Centigrade while at sea level. But as 'calorie' is so widely adopted, I'll use it when discussing energy intake and expenditure.

disappeared from the world, and the consequences. Blair was the lead editor of a landmark 1996 report by the US Surgeon General into activity levels, which kicked off much of the modern era of government guidelines on the subject.[8] He is also, incidentally, one of the pioneers of the idea that it is far better for your health to be overweight and active, rather than slim and immobile, which we'll hear more about later.

Blair is now aged eighty, old enough to remember first-hand how much things have changed in the home. 'Do you want me to tell you who is the real cause of all of these problems?' he tells me, his voice crackling with energy and mischief down the phone. 'It was James Watt, inventing that steam engine. But to be serious, we've been engineering human energy expenditure down and down. I grew up on a farm in Kansas, and I didn't have to do any exercise. I worked my tail off. At 5:30am Daddy would make me go out and get those cows in, and milk them, and feed them, and work all day. Thank goodness I did go to school, so there were a few hours during the school year when I didn't have to be out there.

'I remember when my grandma got a vacuum cleaner. I think it was 1944. And when my parents got electricity out on the farm, I didn't have to carry all those logs in for Mom to put on the stove to cook dinner. On and on and on we've engineered human energy expenditure, down and down and down. I'm not saying we shouldn't have these modern, wonderful devices, but what it means is, we've got to find ways for people to build a little more activity back into their lives.'[9]

A world immobile

Seven-plus decades on from the Blair family's first vacuum cleaner, how inactive are we as a species? The short answer is:

very – and probably even more so than even the official statistics indicate.

The long-standing way for academics to assess activity levels has been to use questionnaires. But as Blair or any other researcher of a similar vintage will resignedly tell you, people cannot always be trusted. My favourite summary comes from James Skinner, a now-retired professor of exercise science at Arizona State University, who once wrote, wisely: 'As a general rule, people overestimate what they do, and underestimate what they eat.' Skinner cited a US study in which people were asked to name which sports they took part in. Even allowing for some of them engaging in more than one sport, the number of people who reported doing just the top ten activities was greater than the entire population of the United States.[10]

Directly monitoring individual movements is now far easier, thanks to the advent of electronic activity tracking, familiar to anyone who has browsed the step count statistics on their smartphone. Many studies now use tiny, Bluetooth-connectable devices, which can feed researchers 24-hour flows of data about every movement and rest, however small or brief. I managed to borrow one of these research-grade devices to track my own activity levels, with eye-opening results, as we'll see later in the book. All that said, when it comes to population-wide studies, especially ones comparing countries, much of the information still tends to be based on surveys and questionnaires. As such, however gloomy the global activity averages, it should be remembered that things are probably worse in real life.

When researchers investigate whether people are considered inactive, thus risking their long-term health, the standard metric is failing to reach at least 150 minutes a week of moderately intensive activity, or 75 minutes of vigorous activity, ideally spread out over five or so days and in bouts of at least ten minutes. The precise definitions of moderate and intense are slightly complex, and I will detail them in the next chapter. But there are countless lists of suggested activities which give a good general idea. For example, moderate activity covers things like walking at a brisk pace, and more strenuous housework chores such as vacuuming, and gardening. To reach intense exertion levels you need to be running, or cycling fairly quickly, or doing difficult manual work like digging a ditch.

This 150-minute gauge has become more or less universal, and is used by the World Health Organization (WHO), Public Health England (PHE) and the US Department of Health, among others. It must be remembered that this is just a minimum level seen as necessary to maintain health, and yet many millions of people don't get anywhere near it. The latest figures for England show that for adults, 66 per cent of men and 58 per cent of women meet these guidelines.[11] This is, however, only part of the story. A more recent but now equally ubiquitous global recommendation from PHE, the WHO and others is that to preserve bone strength and prevent muscle wastage as people age, adults should do some sort of strength-based activity twice a week, whether lifting weights or something like carrying heavy shopping. When the requirements for both aerobic and muscular activity are taken into account, the proportion of people who reach the minimum falls to 31 per cent of men and 23 per cent of women.[12]

The picture gets notably worse when it comes to children. They should aim for an hour of moderate-to-vigorous activity every single day, with those aged under five active for at least three hours daily. In fact, the UK guidance for the latter age group says children so young should never be immobile for long periods, apart from when they're asleep. But in the UK, only 22 per cent of those aged five to fifteen are reaching the minimum, a figure that declines below 15 per cent in adolescence.

Even worse are the statistics for the youngest children, aged two to four, whose mandated three hours a day of movement is vital to lay down bone density and build muscles, as well as acquire the motor skills needed for life. Just 9 per cent manage this.[13]

The UK is no outlier. In fact, in global terms it is broadly typical. Just over a week before the opening of the 2012 London Olympics, revered medical journal *The Lancet* devoted an issue to what it described as the worldwide 'pandemic of physical inactivity'. While the edition was timed to coincide with a sporting event, the stress was very much on everyday activity. 'It is not about running on a treadmill, whilst staring at a mirror and listening to your iPod,' the *Lancet* editors wrote in an introduction. 'It is about using the body that we have in the way it was designed, which is to walk often, run sometimes, and move in ways where we physically exert ourselves regularly, whether that is at work, at home, in transport to and from places, or during leisure time in our daily lives.'[14]

Among the papers was a study by a team of academics seeking to quantify for the first time the global extent of inactive lifestyles. Led by Pedro Hallal, a Brazilian epidemiologist, it took data from just under 90 per cent of the world's population, using a recently agreed standardised international physical activity questionnaire, allowing for the first time robust comparisons between countries and regions.

The headline figure was that 31.1 per cent of people aged fifteen or older were insufficiently active. For those aged thirteen to fifteen, four in five across the world were not meeting the targets.

The study also uncovered the sheer variation across regions, countries, genders and ages. While 43 per cent of adults were inactive in the Americas, this fell to 17 per cent in southeast Asia. Between individual nations the difference was more extreme still, going from fewer than 5 per cent of people not meeting activity guidelines in Bangladesh to very nearly 80 per cent in Malta, the Mediterranean island which despite its idyllic holiday destinations is dominated by car travel. Globally, women were less active than men – 34 per cent were too immobile against 28 per cent – and older people tended to perform less well.[15]

Another huge international project has sought to specifically chart the activity levels of children and teenagers. The somewhat ponderously named Global Matrix 3.0 Physical Activity Report Card covers forty-nine countries, and is regularly updated. Fittingly for a study involving young people, each country's results are given in a school report–style grading system of A to F. To extend the parallel a little further, it's fair to say that if many nations were handed such a report at school, they'd probably try to lose it on the way home, or quietly feed it to the dog.

Countries are rated both for overall youth activity levels, and for specifics such as organised school sport, active travel and input from government. The column for overall grades is a pretty sorry one, featuring a handful of Fs – hang your heads in shame, China, Belgium, Scotland and South Korea – and a mass of Ds, with the USA and Australia both awarded a D-minus. England scrapes a C-minus, with poor scores for active travel and sitting time redeemed in part by school sports.

The only country to gain above a C is Slovenia, topping the table with a highly respectable overall A-minus. The small and mountainous former Yugoslav state might be a geographical minnow – the world's 150th biggest country by size, it has a population of just 2 million – but is keenly studied by those interested in population-wide physical activity, and we shall return to it later in the book.[16]

Yet another international study has examined a series of countries to firstly assess how much worse inactivity levels have become in recent decades, and then extrapolate current trends to see what might be coming in future decades. It makes the assessment using a bespoke health metric which the US researchers titled, *Sleep, Leisure, Occupation, Transportation, and Home-based Activities*. This gives you the acronym *SLOTH*, something I can only imagine brought a self-satisfied chuckle to whoever first coined it.

In the UK, the project found, overall activity levels had fallen 20 per cent in just over three decades, with the amount of exertion people undergo in their work dropping by almost half. By 2030, the researchers predicted, total activity for Britons will be 35 per cent lower than in the mid-1960s. In China, average activity is expected to fall notably more quickly, by a half between the early 1990s and 2030. It is, however, the US where the most astonishing figures lurked. The academics calculated that on current trends, by 2030 the average American will, over an average week, expend only about 15 per cent more total bodily energy than someone who spent the entire seven days in bed.[17] If that sounds worrying, it should be.

The myth of personal choice

In the 2008 Pixar film *WALL·E*, while the eponymous solitary robot endlessly cleans up a rubbish-ruined Earth, the people of the twenty-ninth century are portrayed as space-dwelling, corpulent, jumpsuit-dressed adult-babies, who spend their lives on mobile reclining chairs, a screen permanently at hand. It can be difficult to read studies about the seemingly unstoppable decline in human movement without viewing the film as prophetic, as well as an indictment of humanity's collective decision to slide towards a future of indolence, lethargy and pharmaceutically managed ill-health.

But such a judgemental stance is a grave mistake. The decline in physical activity has had many drivers, but a sudden, global outbreak of idleness is not one of them. This is a crucial point to stress. In fact, one of the reasons the crisis has advanced, largely unchecked, for so long is because governments have ducked responsibility by falsely portraying the issues as based on individual choice and willpower.

This is a complex area, and worth exploring properly. To begin with, it is true that most people, if prompted, probably have at least a basic idea that moving more and sitting less is, on balance, likely to be better for their health. A lot will have heard about the 150-minutes-a-week activity target. Even more will most likely know another much-pushed goal, that of walking 10,000 steps a day. So why do so few people manage it?

One idea that often gets mentioned is insufficient time. It is true that for all the predictions of automation ushering in a life of leisure, many people work just as many hours, or more, than their parents did a few decades earlier. This theory, however, comes with a fairly big caveat. In the words of William Haskell, a now-retired Stanford University professor who is one of the founding figures of the modern physical activity world: 'Surveys show that the most frequent given reason for not being more physically active is lack of time, but this is in a population that reports at least several hours of TV-watching each day.'[18]

Haskell is being a touch mischievous. Watching television is a leisure pursuit, often done in the evening alongside family or other loved ones. It can take significant gumption to wave away the proffered glass of wine, peel yourself from the sofa and head out for a run, or to the gym. This is what public health experts like to call 'discretionary time'. Carving out chunks from it can be a big ask.

This is the central point: if you really want physical movement to embed in someone's life, it has to be in the form of another beloved public health term – 'incidental activity'. This is, at its simplest, activity which takes place almost as an afterthought, because it forms part of your regular day. It is what happened in the past when people did farm chores, or carried in wood for the fire, or walked to school. This was just life. In contrast, sport and exercise generally happen in discretionary time, which is one of the main reasons they are so unsuited to replacing regular exertion as a population-wide driver of better health.

The distinction between these two very different things is often missed, not least by governments. In the broadest terms, physical activity is every single piece of movement you make during the day, from brushing your teeth in the morning, to walking up a flight of stairs to your office, or sprinting to catch a train. Exercise is just a subset of physical activity. It is activity which, to use one formal, academic definition, is 'planned, structured, repetitive, and purposive in the sense that improvement or maintenance of one or more components of physical fitness is an objective'.[19]

If that isn't completely clear, take an example from my own life. I'm currently writing this book in an empty flat about three miles from where I live in south London, borrowed as a short-term writing base. This morning, like more or less every time I have made the trip, I cycled. This was very much physical activity, but not exercise – I did it primarily because it was by far the quickest and most convenient way to travel. Yes, according to a wrist-worn fitness monitor I have borrowed for self-experiment purposes while writing the book, I expended around 170 calories and pushed my heart rate to a peak of 151 beats per minute. But the exertion came about as a side effect, not a primary intention, even if the health benefits were, for me, both known and welcome. Instead, if I had decided to take a day off from the laptop, put on some bike clothes and ridden a few miles further south into the green belt countryside before returning home, this would also have been activity, but exercise as well.

My example highlights something else. The route is almost all on roads without any protected bike lanes. So, in deciding to cycle, I had to make the conscious choice for my unprotected body to directly share road space with two-tonne slabs of metal, gliding closely past me, even at relatively low speeds of around 30mph. I'm okay with doing this because I've cycled alongside cars for years, and I more or less know what to expect. I'm also male and in middle age, one of the demographics more likely to brave urban streets on a bike. But many other people would not be so bullish. And so travelling by bike, the method through which I gain a significant proportion of my weekly physical activity, would be entirely closed off to them.

This is a vital point to consider in our story of vanishing everyday movement – it is a far broader issue than slightly trite discussions about personal responsibility. As soon as you start examining the world from the perspective of adding activity into your routine, you quickly see how thoroughly, how carefully, and at times how cunningly the built environment that surrounds us has been redesigned over the past seventy or so years to make regular exertion an increasingly difficult, at times almost impossible, choice.

To take another example, think about the last time you walked into an office block or large hotel. Almost certainly, the lifts would have been in direct view. But the stairs? If you wanted to climb even a single flight you would probably have had to hunt along a corridor for the recessed fire door, made sure you didn't set off an alarm in opening it, and then trekked up a generally blank, narrow, windowless stairwell in the hope you could open the door at your destination. It's not exactly intuitive.

The disincentives to movement exist in just about every environment in which we live our lives, and come in many forms. If you have a desk-based job, then if email reduced the number of times you walked twenty yards down the office to talk to a colleague, then the recent plethora of text-based chat apps might have stopped this altogether. Meanwhile, the rise of online retailers has played a significant role in the ebbing away of that most basic of leisure-time physical actions, walking round the shops. As soon as you start thinking in this way, the examples crop up in virtually every part of life.

I discussed all this with Xand van Tulleken, a British doctor who has a master's degree in public health but is primarily known as a TV presenter on medical and health matters, often alongside his identical twin and fellow doctor, Chris.

One of the main parts of van Tulleken's job is to explain often complex health ideas to mass audiences, and he is very eloquent on why people's choices in areas such as being active are nowhere near as straightforward as they might seem. 'One of the things I often end up saying to people is that the only person who can really affect your health is you,' he tells me. 'And that is true as individuals. We are just making all the choices that determine our life expectancy. But we're making them in an environment where we are unbelievably constrained.'

Van Tulleken notes that living, as he does, in a relatively privileged stratum of society where virtually no one smokes or drinks to excess and most exercise regularly can bring a temptation to feel, as he puts it, 'slightly smug'. He warns against such feelings: 'Really, that's bollocks. You would have to go a long way in the UK to find someone who sincerely didn't know that beer was bad, fags were bad, or exercise was good. But for some people it's made enormously difficult.

'I am not an exemplar of a healthy life by any means. But if

I had two jobs, was a single parent trying to support kids with special needs, with an uncertain future myself, I would find it very, very much harder not to eat terrible food and seek joy in unhealthy things. If I think about how hard it is for me to make a good choice, and then imagine stripping away my safety nets, my parachutes, I think it would be so difficult.'[20]

Sport won't change things

Van Tulleken describes this prevailing narrative about physical activity as 'the cult of individual responsibility'. This illusion is sustained in no small part by the parallel commodification of exercise, represented as something theoretically available to all but, in practice, often impossible for those poor in money or time, or otherwise challenged. It is illuminating to consider how the decades-long drift away from everyday movement has been so closely tracked by the gradual evolution of sport and gym-going into a value-laden semi-religion, with bodily health viewed not as a routine occurrence but a personal project, one closely attached to appearance, status and wealth.

While the idea of gymnasiums comes from the Ancient Greeks, the arrival of their modern equivalents coincided, both chronologically and geographically, with the initial peaks of industrialisation and urbanisation, just as centuries of every-day movement started to gradually ebb away. The first modern gyms were associated with the curious and relatively short-lived phenomenon of Muscular Christianity, a movement based on faith-based masculine athleticism which grew out of the English public school system in the 1850s. It later took root in the US and the associated movement of the YMCA, where it was respon-sible for the invention of basketball and volleyball.

As the decades progressed, the modern cult of exercise began to emerge. In a fascinating book about the fitness industry,[21] Jennifer Smith Maguire, a British-based academic who specialises in the sociology of consumer culture, points out that celebrity personal trainers are by no means a new phenomenon. In the 1920s, Artie McGovern, a former flyweight boxer who ran a New York gym, became the must-have physical guru for Broadway stars and Wall Street financiers alike, after helping the overweight and overindulging Babe Ruth recover from a trough in his baseball career. It was around the same time that Angelo Siciliano, a somewhat scrawny Italian immigrant to the US, but now beefed up, rebranded himself as Charles Atlas, making a fortune selling exercise regimes based around newspaper adverts in which bullies kicked sand into the face of young weaklings.

The growth of the modern gym-as-personal-temple is more recent, with Smith Maguire identifying the turning point as 1975, when the New York City Yellow Pages replaced its listings for 'gymnasiums' with the new category of 'health clubs'. The boom since then has been staggering. It can be difficult to quantify, but various estimates put the worldwide annual revenues of the health club and fitness industry at about £65 billion, significantly more than the GDP of countries like Bulgaria and Croatia.[22]

We now have a glaring divide of physicality. On the one side are the minority of adherents to the exercise industry, where running shoes can cost £200 and yoga mats even more, and where new fads arrive with tech industry–like rapidity. Consider Peloton, a US start-up offering spin classes streamed to your home, using a £2,000 stationary bike. It was launched in 2013 with a few hundred thousand pounds gathered from a crowd-funding website. Six years later, an initial share offering valued the company at £6.5 billion.[23]

Another phenomenon is the tendency of some people towards

ever-greater levels of exertion. Ultrarunning is any event where the route is longer than the 26-and-a-bit miles of a marathon, although they often span 50 or 100 miles, or greater. These are far from new, but until the past few years they tended to be rare and extremely niche events. Not anymore. In the UK alone, there are now about 500 such events a year, a ten-fold increase in just a decade.[24]

Even as overall activity levels stagnate, the UK now has an estimated 10 million people who are members of a gym, a 25 per cent increase in the past five years.[25] Modern gyms in particular epitomise this increasingly elitist approach to exertion. 'It's not just about exercise, or about how muscles are looking a certain way,' Smith Maguire tells me. 'There's a whole moral economy around how you approach yourself as a site of work, as a site of display for others, as a place for working out your identity.'[26]

A couple of years ago, when the high-end US gym chain Equinox opened a new £350-a-month outlet in St James's, one of central London's most expensive mini-enclaves, Harvey Spevak, the company's executive chairman, gave an interview to the *Financial Times*[27] which could have been explicitly designed to illustrate Smith Maguire's points. Equinox gyms' patrons, Spevak said, were not the sort to be satisfied with two visits a week – more like two classes every day. 'They want it all,' Spevak told the interviewer with almost paternal pride. 'They want to figure out a way they can feel good, look good, be active, and be with like-minded individuals as well as thrive in whatever their personal objectives are.' Equinox also has a parallel chain of five-star hotels, intended for what Spevak called, somewhat intimidatingly, the 'high-performance traveller'.

All this can be hugely excluding. Even lower-cost, mass-market gyms, some of which have made admirable attempts to reach out to a broader market, can remain intimidating environments to many. Smith Maguire is highly sceptical about gyms of any sort making real inroads into overall inactivity levels. 'The commercial fitness industry itself is a product of that draining away of everyday activity. Markets rely on problems,' she says. 'I'm deeply suspicious of any health promotion strategy that rests on individuals making specific choices, because those choices are not individually theirs to make.'

Numerous governments have bought into the illusion that urging people to exercise in their spare time can make up for reduced activity in everyday life. The UK is something of a poster child for this approach. Recent decades have seen minimal investment in areas such as infrastructure for safer walking and cycling. But at the same time, the amount of public money put into elite sport has grown vastly. At the 1996 Atlanta Olympics, the UK squad, assembled on a total budget of about £5 million, came thirty-eighth in the medal table. This prompted an outpouring of national angst, followed by an inflow of money from National Lottery funds. By the Sydney Olympics four years later, the UK team's budget was nearly £59 million. For Rio in 2016, with the UK now second in the medals tally, this had reached £274 million.[28] Coincidentally, the Rio budget is almost exactly the same as annual government spending on Public Health England,[29] which is not only tasked with promoting more activity, but also leads on efforts in areas including tobacco and alcohol, as well as, of course, infectious diseases like coronavirus. This is all about to change, after the government announced it will replace PHE with a new organisation focused on infectious illnesses, with the preventative health work hived off elsewhere, possibly to local government.

Those millions spent on Olympic medals might have brought a few weeks of national cheer, but there is minimal evidence they boosted overall activity levels, whether in sport or elsewhere. Statistics from Sport England, the same body responsible for handing out the Olympic money, show that the proportion of people who say they never take part in any sport – about 55 per cent of the population – has stayed more or less static for a decade.[30]

A particularly telling example is cycling. After British cyclists won dozens of gold medals over a succession of Olympics, and then took a series of Tour de France titles, there was much talk of a boom in cycling numbers. And for a period there was a rise in bike sales, and an increase in cycle commuter numbers in a handful of places. But if you look at the detailed statistics, any impression of real change evaporates. Government figures show that from 2002 to 2018, the average number of bike trips per person per year stayed largely flat, declining marginally from an already minuscule eighteen to seventeen. The average number of miles ridden did rise a bit, which was perhaps the one impact of all the new racing cyclists – they tended to go for slightly longer rides.[31]

Another problem with sport is that its benefits are not felt evenly. People from disadvantaged socio-economic groups have long been less likely to participate in physical activity overall, and this effect is magnified with exercise. The most recent UK data shows that while 51 per cent of people in the top social grades as defined in government statistics take part in at least some sport, for those in the most deprived groups this drops to 35 per cent.[32]

Prompted by decades of government messaging, many people try exercise and then find that an initial burst of enthusiasm gradually evaporates. Insiders from the fitness industry will happily tell you that a significant part of the business model of most gyms are the clients known as 'sleepers' – those who take out a membership but then rarely, if ever, attend. There are varying statistics for absentee members, but one seemingly rigorous 2017

UK poll suggested that 11 per cent of people had not removed their gym cards from their wallets once in the past year.[33]

There is deep concern among many public health professionals that the focus on sport rather than more regular movement allows governments to pretend they are tackling inactivity, and ignore the wider problems. Dr Adrian Davies, whom we heard from in the last chapter, is particularly scathing about what he calls the 'Eton playing fields mindset', saying: 'There's nothing wrong with sport, but if you look at the fitness levels of the whole population, we need to do routine, moderate physical activity before you start to ask people to engage in vigorous activity.'[34]

Additionally, the glaring contrast between Harvey Spevak's small minority of toned, have-it-all, twice-a-day gym-goers and the four-in-ten Britons who barely exert their bodies at all is fertile ground for shame and stigma, particularly when excess weight is involved. Such judgements are deeply unfair.

This is one of the most vital messages I would hope people take from this book: labelling someone who is inactive as lazy and ignorant, or to condemn yourself in those terms, is to utterly miss the point. This is a process which has played out across whole populations, and over decades. This is not an individual story, or a failure of willpower. It is much, much bigger than that.

Next steps:

Think about your routine, and how and when you are physical. Is it just through exercise – and if so, can it be hard to find the time? Then think about how you might be able to incorporate any sort of exertion into everyday life – everything from climbing one flight of stairs to parking 200 metres further away than normal – instead.

2

The Miracle Pill: Small Doses Have Big Impacts

Dr Richard Mackenzie knows more than most people about the ways activity can affect the human body. He has worked with elite cyclists, and in the laboratory where the former marathon world record holder Paula Radcliffe had her fitness tested. His current research examines how a lack of movement can make people intolerant to insulin, and thus develop type 2 diabetes, one of the most prevalent, destructive and medically costly chronic conditions of the modern era. A lot of his work involves using isotopes, adapted elements which can be easily traced through the body to try to see the effects of activity at a cellular level.

But sitting in the student café at Roehampton University in southwest London, a noisy, airy space with decidedly un-London views onto playing fields and then the green expanse of Richmond Park in the distance, Mackenzie is cheerfully honest about how much he has so far discovered about these biological fundamentals. 'Almost nothing,' he laughs. 'Unless you're a grant-awarding body, and I'll tell you a very different story.' The science is, he says, 'very challenging – even the whole-body level isn't really understood'.

Mackenzie is perhaps being unduly modest, given the potential future benefits of his research. One strand examines how certain proteins might act as what he calls 'a negative feedback loop' to push people into type 2 diabetes. This is the lifestyle-related variant of diabetes, distinct from type 1, which is a lifelong autoimmune condition. Type 2 diabetes begins when the tissues in someone's body stop responding properly to insulin, the hormone central to the maintenance of healthy blood sugar levels, putting them into what is called pre-diabetes. Mackenzie's efforts focus on how some people with pre-diabetes then move to the full-blown condition, with the ensuing regime of medication and possible serious complications, and others do not. He has recruited a test group of pre-diabetic people with the hope of observing various protein interactions which then cause one or the other outcome. The eventual aim, which Mackenzie concedes is 'a long way off', could be some form of bespoke treatment based around the metabolic profile of individual patients.

Other studies led by Mackenzie examine how activity reverses the diabetic starting point. This involves taking a volunteer and infusing them with higher-than-usual levels of insulin to mimic the effects of pre-diabetes, balanced with a careful counter-dose of glucose to make sure they don't slip into a diabetic coma. 'You might laugh,' Mackenzie says as he explains this to me. 'But we do make sure no one is harmed.'

Once this artificial pre-diabetic state is induced, the subject starts exercising, and Mackenzie and his team observe the way activity improves their body's ability to process glucose. I ask him how long it takes – a few hours, perhaps a day? He replies with a smile: 'You can see the effects begin within seconds. It's that quick. The subjects can become pre-diabetic, if you like, and then revert to healthy before they leave the lab.'

It is not only the timescale which is exaggeratedly tiny – so is the range of movement needed to have a metabolic effect. Mackenzie explains: 'As we're infusing the insulin, even modest things like giggling, using muscles that allow you to laugh, mean that we have to infuse more glucose because those muscles are responding very well to the insulin. And it always works. There are very, very few people that exercise won't help.'

Cutting-edge studies about the cellular process of glucose intolerance might seem a bit distanced from this book's story of everyday activity. But they illustrate one of the most astonishing aspects of physical movement: for all the harm caused by its absence, more or less the very moment you start to use your body again, it feels the benefits.

For decades, the conventional wisdom was that for activity to have much of a health-restoring effect it had to be at least reasonably vigorous and fairly regular. These ideas are now being rapidly rethought, in part due to the advent of sophisticated electronic activity trackers, like the one I borrowed, which have helped researchers to properly measure limited amounts of low-level movement and follow the health outcomes.

Another emerging consensus dispenses with the assumption that activity has to last a certain period of time, arguing that even the briefest bursts can be beneficial. This is the new, and hopeful, world of inactivity advice. Yes, if you can reach well-known targets like 10,000 steps a day or 150 minutes of activity a week, that's great. But in terms of both amount and intensity, just about anything is better than nothing at all.

Making yourself younger

So why does the human body respond so well to movement – and, in turn, so badly to prolonged periods of immobility? Let's start with a slightly oblique approach. How do we even know for certain that, as humans, we are intended to be active? This question is tackled in one of the best, and heaviest, of the many activity physiology textbooks I acquired for my research. At the start of the first chapter of the breezeblock-size *Physical Activity and Health*, it is posed by Professor Claude Bouchard, a venerable and now largely retired US activity expert who led the book's equally heavyweight editorial team.

Bouchard's answer comes in three parts, and I was immediately struck by its elegance. First of all, he says, the body is clearly well adapted to exertion, given that healthy adults are able to increase their resting metabolic rate ten-fold or more, and maintain this state for a considerable period of time. Secondly, he notes in a convincing if somewhat circular answer, we know the body is meant to move on a daily basis because of the range and extent of ill-health that follows if it does not. Finally – and here I slightly précis Bouchard's more sober academic style – while we modern humans have created an environment in which we can, if we choose, permanently lounge amid a sedentary haze of car travel, home-delivered food and social interaction via a pocket-sized screen, our early ancestors were clearly dependent for survival on regular physical exertion, meaning it is demonstrably inherent to our evolution.[1]

In the same way as this book is not intended to be a step-by-step guide to better health, it is definitely not a physiology textbook. But for me to explain why regular physical movement is so fundamental to human wellbeing I need to outline a few principles about how it affects the body, and what happens when it is not there.

To begin with the utter basics, energy is expended every time we move. I'm currently sitting down to write this chapter. Yes, this is not ideal for long periods, as we'll see later in the book. In a few minutes I plan to get up and make a cup of tea. When I do that, a much more significant selection of my skeletal muscles than are now being used to sit and type will spring, or in some cases creak, into action. Skeletal muscle is the biggest mass of tissue in the human body, comprising more than 600 individual muscles. It's also the only type of muscle we control consciously. The others are cardiac muscle, which, as the name suggests, is found in the heart, and smooth muscle, located mainly in organs like the stomach and intestine.

When I get up from the chair and march the six or seven paces from my desk to the compact kitchen of my temporary writing flat, my muscles will be powered by a molecule called adenosine triphosphate, or ATP. This is not a storage for energy, like carbohydrates. ATP is often described as the 'currency unit' of energy transfer. Specifically, ATP provides the energy for myosin, a motor protein, to bind to actin, another protein, pulling the actin in, thus shortening muscle fibres. For my imminent mission to the kitchen, these will principally be in my legs, the location of some of the biggest muscles in the body, where the ATP will be converted into adenosine diphosphate (ADP) or adenosine monophosphate (AMP). While I stand waiting for the kettle to boil, my ATP will be replenished by aerobic respiration, using inhaled oxygen.

But if, hypothetically, I interrupted the tea making to dash out of the front door and run up and down the short if fairly steep hill outside until I was completely out of breath, the ATP would be replaced using the different, notably more short-term, chemical process of anaerobic respiration. This also produces lactate, which is in itself not a problem for the body, but also tends to increase acidity, and in turn the burning feeling known only too well to even recreational athletes, which would before long make my legs ache, and prompt me to come to a wheezing halt. The muscle-aching substance is traditionally known as 'lactic acid', but these days scientists like to distinguish between the lactate, which is generally benign, and the acidity, which is not.

That's the mechanics, or rather the chemistry and biology. So why is a habitually immobile life, or at least one mainly devoid of moderate exertion, so bad for you? One of the apparent main factors comes back to ATP. It is produced by mitochondria, a sub-part of individual cells that is generally described as their 'engine unit'. Mitochondria tend to work less well as we age, but this also happens with prolonged inactivity.

Sluggish mitochondria are bad health news for all sorts of reasons. They are particularly important in the heart, due to the constant energy expended there. Numerous studies have linked poorly functioning mitochondria to all sorts of cardiovascular diseases, including furred arteries, high blood pressure and heart attacks. Mitochondrial dysfunction is also seen as increasing the risk of type 2 diabetes, and is implicated in the cellular mutations that can lead to cancer.

The good news is how rapidly this process can seemingly be reversed through movement. One 2017 US study put groups of volunteers through various twelve-week exercise regimes. Half the participants were young, under thirty, and the others were aged between sixty-five and eighty. At the end of the process, the younger group had increased their mitochondrial capacity by no less than 49 per cent. For the older participants, the gain was an even more impressive 69 per cent.[2]

If such results lead you to think that physical activity can slow the ageing process, you're perhaps more correct than you realised. Other studies have examined its effect on telomeres, tiny sequences of molecules that effectively act as a cap on chromosomes, shielding them. Elizabeth Blackburn, an Australian scientist who won a Nobel Prize for her work on telomeres, describes them elegantly by saying that if you think of your chromosomes as shoelaces, telomeres are 'the little protective tips at the end'.[3] If telomeres wear down, this can cause cell malfunction and all sorts of diseases associated with ageing. The shortening of telomeres happens with age anyway, but also because of lifestyle factors including a poor diet, lack of sleep and, particularly, inactive living.

One particularly striking recent study examined telomere length in nearly 6,000 Americans of various ages and activity levels. It found that the most active people were on average nine years younger by telomere length than those who were completely sedentary.[4] Nine years. It's a repeated refrain of this book, but just imagine the universal acclaim if you could package that effect into a tablet.

Zooming out a little from this cellular focus, another reason physical activity is so vital is because of the role skeletal muscle plays in human health. It has only been established fairly recently that, rather than being what you might call a neutral force in the body, skeletal muscle is part of the endocrine system, the hormone-producing function associated mainly with glands like the pituitary and thyroid. Muscles secrete not just hormones, but also cytokines, a type of amino acid chain which helps regulate the body's immune response, and which can prompt inflammation. Studies have shown that a lack of regular movement can unbalance these substances, and assist what one paper called the 'vicious circle' of muscle wastage, extra fat, and then the development of all sorts of diseases.

Any accumulation of fat – or, to use its posh name, adipose tissue – in itself also brings complications, because fat is also now known to be part of the endocrine system, and has a role in the secretion and synthesis of various hormones, some affecting sensitivity to insulin, and thus linked to type 2 diabetes.

These effects happen over time, but as we saw at the start of the chapter, movement has a more-or-less immediate impact on how the body functions. At the centre of this acute response to movement are lipoproteins, particles which transport various types of fat around your bloodstream, including cholesterol and less household-name fats like triglycerides.

In the broadest terms, while some blood-fats are seen as unproblematic, like high-density lipoprotein cholesterol (HDL), significant levels of another type of cholesterol, low-density lipoprotein (LDL), and of triglycerides spell trouble, and are linked to an increased risk of heart disease, not least via constricted arteries. It has been shown conclusively that activity shifts the balance of these substances away from the health-harming variants.

Many dozens of studies have proved this effect, some showing that even walking on a treadmill can help notably reduce lipaemia, the technical term for high fat concentrations in the blood.[5] This effect is more significant in people who are otherwise fit, but still happens if you are not.

The other hugely significant function kickstarted by movement is the processing of sugars in our bloodstream, a vital ability in the prevention of type 2 diabetes and other metabolic disorders. Skeletal muscle plays a key role in this, and as we saw with Richard Mackenzie's experiments, even a single bout of activity can improve the body's response to insulin.

The role of movement in helping us deal with both fats and sugars is particularly important in the immediate aftermath of food, what is known officially as the postprandial state. There is, of course, one problem here. In the modern world, most people consume their largest single dose of high-fat, high-sugar foods in their evening meal. And then, rather than going out for a bracing stroll, they instead walk just a few paces to the sofa – if they're not there already – and watch TV for a couple of hours. It's no wonder our bodies eventually protest.

A body shut down

I ask Xand van Tulleken, the public health expert and TV doctor we heard from earlier, how he explains the health dangers of long-term inactivity to people in the most basic terms. He makes the parallel with space travel, and the well-documented impact on astronauts' bodies of zero gravity and the ensuing lack of physical exertion, including weaker bones, wasted muscles, and even longer-term changes.

It is an intriguing parallel. As mentioned before, Van Tulleken is one of a pair of identical twins. Perhaps the most fascinating study on the health effects of space travel saw NASA compare the changes to Scott Kelly, an astronaut who spent six months on board the International Space Station, and his identical twin, Mark, who remained on Earth. As well as changes to muscle mass and bone density, the NASA scientists found Scott Kelly experienced narrowing of his arteries, while his brother did not. Perhaps most unexpectedly, the long space flight appeared to alter some of his genes, particularly those connected to the immune system, with not all the changes reversed when he returned to normal gravity.[6]

Another parallel van Tulleken uses is what happens to people left immobile in hospital. 'If I put you in intensive care you will lose about 2–3 per cent of your muscle mass per day because you're still,' he explains. 'And that's what we're all bloody doing at home now. What I try to explain to people is that when you don't move your body it starts to just decay immediately. It's very expensive for your body to maintain itself the way it is. And so as soon as there's no stress put on your body, it's like, "Well, fuck this, I'm just going to shut it all down." Over time, what it will do is increase your risk of every single illness and it will make you die earlier, and along the way, your life will become much worse.'[7]

This might be a more vivid summary of the risks from inactivity than found in the official guidance, but the core message of both is the same. One of the most comprehensive government round-ups of the relevant science comes in the Physical Activity Guidelines Advisory Committee, or PACAG, a near-800-page report to the US government by a panel of the great and good of the physical activity world.[8]

First published in 2008 and updated ten years later, it stresses the 'clear inverse dose–response relationship between the amount of moderate-to-vigorous physical activity and all-cause mortality'. In other words, if you don't move about much, your chances of dying before your time are increased. The 2008 edition put this effect at about 30 per cent. The 2018 update dispensed with the specific figure, but added that 'the strength of the evidence is very unlikely to be modified by more studies of these outcomes'. In other words: case closed.

There are many hundreds of individual studies purely on the risk of an earlier death from long-term inactivity, all reaching pretty much the same conclusion via slightly different routes. One mammoth piece of research which tracked the lives of more than 250,000 Americans aged fifty-plus found that those who reached the recommended minimum of 150 minutes a week of moderate activity had a 27 per cent lower chance of dying over the five-year research period than those who were inactive. If they managed at least some vigorous exertion, the figure rose to 32 per cent, and for people who managed both, it shot up to 50 per cent. Even engaging in some activity, but below the minimum, reduced the risks by 18 per cent.[9]

Another paper assessed the actual fitness of more than 13,000 men and women, as an objectively measurable proxy for movement. This found that after adjusting for all other factors, among men, those in the least fit 20 per cent of the cohort were more than three times more likely to die over the course of the study than the fittest 20 per cent. With women, the difference between the groups rose to four times.[10]

There are many dozens more such studies, and detailing any more runs the risk of both repetition and gloominess. But it's worth explaining how this risk plays out on a global, population-wide level. One of the main studies in the edition of *The Lancet* devoted to physical inactivity, mentioned in the previous chapter, tried to undertake the most comprehensive reckoning yet of the global burden of illness and early death from inactivity. It was led by I-Min Lee, a professor of epidemiology at Harvard University, who is perhaps the world's foremost modern expert on the connection between inactivity and ill-health. Her co-authors also comprised something of an all-star team from the discipline. They included several people whose names crop up elsewhere in the book, among them Steven Blair, who we also encountered in the last chapter, and Pukka Peska, a Finnish doctor who set up what is generally recognised as one of the most successful public health programmes in modern history. These were people who knew what they were talking about.

Their paper used complex formulae to crunch together the prevalence of inactive living around the world, and then the risks this creates, across nations, for a huge range of conditions including heart disease, high blood pressure, strokes, type 2 diabetes, various cancers, bone health, cognitive function and the risk of falls among older people. The headline conclusions were that, worldwide, inactivity is responsible for between 6 per cent and 10 per cent of all these conditions. This leads, the authors said, to around 9 per cent of deaths worldwide, making inactivity as deadly as the far more discussed issues of smoking and obesity.

Using 2008 as the base year for the data, the paper calculated that this meant 5.3 million fatalities due to inactivity, not far short of 15,000 people a day. The authors, however, noted that given the likelihood of even stronger associations between inactivity and disease than factored in the study, plus that much of the activity data was self-reported and thus likely to be exaggerated, 'our estimates are likely to be very conservative'.[11] Quite how conservative remains to be seen – Lee is currently leading an update of the study – but some epidemiologists privately say the real global death toll is likely to be closer to 7 million or 8 million a year.

It's worth noting that a slightly earlier attempt to come up with an annual global death toll for inactivity, from the World Health Organization (WHO), reached a lower, if still alarming, total. The report from the WHO's Global Burden of Disease team concluded that around 3.2 million deaths a year could be attributed to inactivity, less than tobacco use but more than obesity.[12] But in a follow-up article for *The Lancet* in 2013, Lee and some colleagues examined the discrepancy and argued that the WHO's metrics for activity and the risks of mortality were 'unclear' – as close as a scientist ever gets to openly saying, 'I think you'll find that we were right.'[13]

When it comes to research into the individual diseases and conditions worsened by prolonged inactivity, the number of studies runs into the countless thousands. I'll detail some of them in subsequent chapters, but as an introduction to the sheer scale of the health risks involved, here is a condensed list.

Cardiovascular diseases: The very first research connecting inactivity to poor health, published in 1953[14] and about which we'll hear more in the next chapter, looked at the risk from heart attacks. Subsequent research has shown ever-stronger links between immobile living and not just heart-related deaths but conditions like high blood pressure and narrowed arteries. The benefits are all the more so if the activity is vigorous. One huge study found men who ran for an hour or more a week cut their risk of heart disease by 42 per cent, while those who walked briskly for thirty minutes or more a day saw an 18 per cent reduction.[15] A review of the science in the 2018 PACAG report concluded there is 'no lower limit' for risk reduction – that is, even tiny amounts of movement will do good. This is true, it added, whatever your age, gender, weight or race.[16]

Cancer: Dozens of studies have suggested reaching at least minimum recommended activity levels can reduce the risk of colon cancer by 30–40 per cent in both men and women, while women see a reduction in breast cancer risks of around 20–30 per cent. The PACAG report, which devotes a full sixty-five pages to cancer, concludes that as well as these two there is also a strong relationship between activity and a lower risk of bladder cancer, renal cancer, oesophageal cancer, gastric cancer and endometrial cancer, as well as moderate evidence for lung cancer, and some, if limited, evidence connected to cancers of the blood, prostate, pancreas, ovaries, and head and neck.[17]

Precisely how activity limits these risks remains up for debate, and in part depends on the cancer. One possibility for breast cancer is that when women are active this can reduce concentrations of certain hormones linked to the condition. Another apparent link could be the effect of inactivity on mitochondria. Yet another theory draws links between inactive living and excess weight and inflammation, both of which are implicated with higher cancer risks.

Type 2 diabetes: This is a slightly more complex relationship, as the onset of the lifestyle-related version of the chronic metabolic condition is linked very closely to not just lack of movement but excess weight, as well as excessive time sitting down, with the various factors interconnecting. As a headline figure, studies have shown that a combination of greater activity and dietary interventions can cut the risk of type 2 diabetes in susceptible people by about 60 per cent, far greater than the benefit of any drug yet developed.[18]

Bone and joint health: A hugely significant and often neglected health issue. As we saw with the Neolithic hunter-gatherers earlier, bone mass is intimately connected to activity, with strength laid down in childhood and, if we are not careful, ebbing away in later decades. As an indication of the scale of the problem, in England alone, around 250,000 older people are hospitalised a year because of falls, with an estimated 9,000 dying.[19]

Cognitive function and dementia: This is one of the most fast-moving and exciting areas of activity science. Even senior academics who have seen it all in the physical movement world perk up when they talk about this, with good reason. A series of studies have shown regular activity can seemingly not just reduce your chance of developing Alzheimer's or other forms of dementia, but can even reverse some of the memory-sapping effects of ageing. It appears to particularly improve so-called executive functions, those connected to higher-level cognition like planning and task management, with scans showing the relevant parts of the brain can actually increase in size.

Mental health: The idea of movement or exercise having mood-lifting effects, the much-touted 'runners' high', is long-established, and popularly attributed to a rush of endorphins, the body's natural opiates that are primarily there to dull pain. This is in some doubt, not least due to studies showing no apparent match between people's reported mood and measured endorphin levels. Nonetheless, there is robust, repeated evidence that activity both reduces the risk of developing depression, and can help alleviate the symptoms of those who have it, with some studies suggesting a comparable effect to some drug regimes. There has been a similar effect demonstrated for anxiety, and even some studies showing staying active can assist with some of the symptoms of schizophrenia. Finally, there are numerous studies showing regular activity improves our sleep, both in terms of time and quality.

How much is enough?

There is, of course, an important if hopefully obvious caveat to all this: it is all about population-wide outcomes. It is possible for someone to spend their entire adult life never shifting more than a short trudge from an armchair while maintaining an enthusiastic intake of alcohol and tobacco, and still live to be 100. Similarly, someone else could be permanently active and scrupulously abstemious, and expire from a heart attack at forty. However, both would be statistical outliers. If you are inactive and sedentary, you are not necessarily going to become infirm or die younger than you would otherwise have done, or the converse for those whose life is filled with movement. But, all other factors being equal, the chances of this happening become notably greater.

So how much do you need to do to remain healthy? The first thing to look at is how activity and exertion are measured. There are two basic ways. To an extent, both are the domain of researchers and academics, those able to measure exertion levels and energy expenditure. But they are nonetheless hugely useful as a broad guide of what to aim for.

One metric, used mainly in population-level studies, is the physical activity level, or PAL. This is simply the amount of energy a person actually expends over a 24-hour period divided by their so-called basal metabolic rate (BMR) – that is, how much energy their body needs to just tick over in complete immobility. BMR depends on the individual. Men tend to have a higher level than women, due to larger amounts of muscle, while children's rates are higher than those of adults as a proportion of their body size. The totals are nonetheless perhaps more than you might think, and can easily exceed 1,500 calories per day for an adult.

A PAL measuring anything from one to 1.4 is taken to mean someone is completely sedentary, even a hospital patient. Between 1.4 and 1.6 is inactive, for example someone with a desk job who doesn't exercise outside work. From 1.6 to approaching two is deemed active, perhaps a person with a manual job, or a regular gym-goer. From two to 2.4 makes you very active – if your work isn't physical it requires about two hours of exercise per day. And once you get beyond 2.4, you're basically a professional sportsperson.

The other main measure is a gauge of exertion, called the MET, short for metabolic equivalent. One MET is simply the energy you are expending if you sit down and do nothing. This figure then multiplies according to how strenuous an activity is. This is where the value to a layperson comes in. While it depends on the age and fitness of the person performing the task, it's possible to put broad MET figures to everyday activities. Thus, basic housework could be two METs, some light gardening more like three. Gentle cycling could take you five or six, while running tends to be twelve METs or above.

This is hugely useful to know, as one of the golden rules of the health benefits of activity is that it depends in part on the level of exertion. In the most basic terms, if light exertion does some good, the dividends really begin if it is moderate, and they multiply again if things become strenuous. In terms of METs, the general guide is that anything less than three METs is light, three to six is moderate, and above six is strenuous.

It is here that we enter the more practical world of guidelines. As we saw in the last chapter, in the twenty-five or so years since governments started giving formal advice on the subject, for adults it has coalesced around the figure of 150 minutes of moderate activity a week. The WHO list of possible moderate activities[20] includes brisk walking, gardening, DIY chores like painting, or playing games with children. Another option is to instead undertake at least seventy-five minutes of vigorous activity, for example reasonably quick cycling, running, labour-intensive gardening, or building work like digging a ditch.

With specific activities, there has been a lot of focus on walking, not least because it's a straightforward thing that virtually everyone does. It is also one of the few areas of movement where a specific target seems to have fully permeated the public consciousness: the magic figure of 10,000 steps a day.

Before we delve into the curious history of that figure, it's worth remembering that for walking to reach the WHO-mandated moderate exertion level, your pace must be 'brisk'. This is often translated to mean about 3mph. However, humans don't have built-in speedometers, and the actual speed will vary depending on factors like height, age and fitness. So what does it mean in more practical terms? I-Min Lee of Harvard University, who led the study into global deaths from inactivity, explains it thus: 'I tend to put it that moderate walking is an intensity where, say, you think about meeting someone for lunch and you're a little bit late so you walk at a pace so you get there in time. Or you can think of it as an intensity level where you can still talk but you can't sing.'[21]

This area is the particular specialisation of Catrine Tudor-Locke, professor of public health at the University of Massachusetts, who is one of the world's foremost experts on the issue of both counting steps and working out how rapid they should be. While she welcomes the way the 10,000-step target has caught on, Tudor-Locke's work focuses increasingly on how to persuade people to walk at sufficient pace. She describes the physical effect of a brisk walk as 'not necessarily sweaty but your heart rate is elevated'.[22]

In one study, Tudor-Locke sought to put precise figures to this. Equal numbers of healthy men and women, split into five-year age groups between twenty-one and forty, were placed on treadmills, with their heart rates measured to see what speed was needed for them to reach moderate exertion. Averaging out the results, Tudor-Locke found that this was a cadence of between 100 and 130 paces per minute.[23] She adds that when people count their steps over a timed minute, many find the 100-step pace 'really quite slow'.

Tudor-Locke explains: 'It's really easy for people to get to moderate intensity. So people say – why are we so worried? It's because in our lives today we very rarely have purposeful walking for any long or persistent amount of time. We might walk from our car park to the office, and that might be the longest walk of the day. That might be a total of eighty steps. You haven't even gotten to 100 steps, let alone 100 steps in a minute.'

This leads to the second part of the equation: how much? It can be a source of some anguish for activity watchers, intensely aware of whether or not they have reached their 10,000-step target. Many people follow this on smartphones, but these measurements are often an approximation. As Tudor-Locke explains: 'Men tend to wear their phones on them, for example in their pocket. But women tend to put their phone in their bag, which they then put down, and walk away from it.' Wrist-worn fitness trackers and smart watches can be more accurate, but even these can be misled. As Tudor-Locke says during our phone call: 'Right now, talking to you, I'm sitting on my butt, but my hands are flailing all around. I'll be getting erroneous steps.'

Does it even matter? The emergence of 10,000 as a step target has a slightly arbitrary history. In the wake of the 1964 Tokyo Olympics, a Japanese company devised and then marketed the first wearable pedometer, the grandfather of all the modern Fitbits. The original advertising shows it looking a bit like an old-fashioned nurse's watch, with a dialled face hanging from a loop you could put on your belt. The key to the device's legacy was its name: the *manpo-kei*, which translates from Japanese as '10,000-step meter'. This is the origin of the target.

It wasn't entirely marketing. The pedometer was devised by a young Japanese researcher, Dr Yoshiro Hatano, who had discovered that Japanese people were averaging only between 3,500 and 5,000 steps a day. His calculation was that boosting it to 10,000 could use up to 20 per cent of a person's caloric intake and thus maintain a healthy weight. And yes, walking 10,000 steps is better than 5,000. But there is an argument that this would have been just as true if Dr Hatano had instead chosen 8,000 steps, or 12,000. Some researchers worry that the endless focus on 10,000 steps might seem a distant goal to the most inactive people, meaning they give up.

Tudor-Locke notes that there can be a benefit in people having an easily remembered number to aim for, like five portions of fruit and vegetables a day, or 150 minutes of activity a week. But in terms of steps, she says, the important message is that everyone should simply try to walk at least a bit more than they do now, and at a slightly quicker pace: 'If you walk further and faster, then the digits take care of themselves.'

Whatever the reasons it was picked as a target, 10,000 steps does seem to be good for you. One recent study followed a large cohort of middle-aged people in the Australian state of Tasmania. It found that over the course of a decade, walking an average of 10,000 steps a day gave a 40 per cent reduced chance of death when compared to those who were largely immobile.[24]

But as new research emerges, orthodoxies about both step amounts and cadence are being challenged. One groundbreaking study, published in 2019, was led, yet again, by the tireless I-Min Lee. It saw more than 16,700 older American women, with an average age of seventy-two, wear electronic step monitors for a week. When their walking data was analysed four years later, by which point 504 had died, the findings were remarkable.

There was, indeed, a relationship between distance and mortality, but it began far lower than 10,000 steps. When the women were put into four groups based on step counts, those in the second lowest of these, with an average of 4,400 a day, had a 41 per cent lower risk of death over the period than those in the bottom quarter, who averaged 2,700. The benefits rose with greater step counts, but seemed to level off at around 7,500 steps a day.

Another apparent anomaly was with the speed. Very few of these women, it is fair to say, could be described as routinely brisk walkers. In the four groups as ranked by step totals, between 93 per cent and 99 per cent of daytime hours were spent either not walking at all, or at a slow amble, up to a maximum of thirty-nine steps a minute – basically, pottering. That left very little time for fairly slow walking of between forty and ninety-nine steps a minute, while 100 steps or more – the supposed baseline for moderate exertion – barely happened at all, making up just 2.2 per cent of the time even among the most active group. And yet the health benefits were still visible.[25]

One possible reason is that exertion is a relative state. Catrine Tudor-Locke's 100-steps-a-minute assessment was based on much younger test subjects, and thus a significantly lower pace could still count as moderate for someone in their seventies. Also, as the study notes, it's also simply possible that for older people the health benefits come as much from just being active at all than necessarily pushing yourself.

This is a new boundary for activity research, Lee says: 'In the past when we said, "You have to do at least moderate-intensity physical activity", that wasn't because we found that light-intensity activity was not beneficial for health, it was because we couldn't measure it well. Now, if you look at some of the recent papers that have come out, we're starting to see that light-intensity activity, which has not been recommended the way moderate- and vigorous-intensity physical activity have, is being shown to be beneficial for health. So I suppose it's been surprising, and now the work is more about reinforcing that any little bit you can do is good for you. And that's encouraging for a lot of people.'

Step counting can still be useful, Lee says, but people don't necessarily have to be fixated on 10,000 a day, especially if they are starting from a low base, and find it intimidating: 'If you are someone who likes to count I would say that as a first goal, for someone who does nothing, try to reach around 4,000 to 5,000 steps. If you're already at that, then 7,000 is a good next step. And if you're at 7,000, then 10,000 is perfect. But, surprisingly, it's a very low level you need to first get at and that's the 4,000- or 5,000-step level. This is for the true couch potatoes.'[26]

Anything is better than nothing

This new era is gradually becoming reflected in the official guidance. A recent initiative devised by Public Health England, called Active Ten, has the very simple goal of trying to get people to walk briskly for ten minutes a day, whether or not it's all in one go. The associated phone app, which monitors whether people have reached the target and politely cajoles them to do so, stresses in very large letters when it first opens that 'every minute counts'.

Similarly, the updated US PACAG guidelines from 2018 note for the first time that if someone is currently inactive, introducing even some light-intensity activity of more or less any type will reduce their risks of developing cardiovascular disease and type 2 diabetes, and of an early death. They also dispense with a previous assessment that bouts of activity should last at least ten minutes, saying any length is beneficial.[27] Yet again, the key is to do something, of more or less any duration.

Another new message public health officials are keen to push is the immediacy of the results. The PACAG report spells it out, saying that on the same day you manage a single session of moderate-to-vigorous physical activity you will see a reduction in blood pressure, better insulin sensitivity, improved sleep, fewer anxiety symptoms, and improved cognitive function. That's not bad for an instant gain.

At the other end of the spectrum, it's worth noting that while there presumably is a maximum dose of activity beyond which the health benefits stop coming, it has not yet been found, even if the dose–response curve does level off and beyond a certain level of extreme activity the health gains can become almost too negligible to measure.

One of the most thorough examinations of this came in a

2016 meta-study comprising almost 150 million person-years of combined scrutiny. The overall conclusion was that while the biggest gains occurred at lower activity levels, their increase remained significant up to pretty Herculean amounts of movement. Using the tally of MET minutes per week – how many METs someone is moving at, multiplied by how many minutes they are doing it, over seven days – it took the standard 150-minute-per-week recommendation for moderate activity to stand for 600 MET minutes, assuming an exertion of four METs. If people managed beyond 600 minutes, they saw significant health gains, which only started to tail off slightly at 3,000 or 4,000 MET minutes per week.

That's between five and nearly seven times more than the minimum recommended amount. The authors helpfully provided a possible timetable for someone to amass even 3,000 MET minutes in a week, and it's fair to say it sounds quite exhausting. The example involves – and remember, this should happen every day of the week – ten minutes of stair climbing, fifteen minutes of vacuuming, gardening for twenty minutes, running for twenty minutes, and walking or cycling for transport for twenty-five minutes. If you did follow this regime, as well as being fit, you would presumably also end up with a well-tended garden and extremely clean carpets.[28]

Another consideration to bear in mind is how often you take your activity, whether gradually over a week, or in one or two short bursts. A fair proportion of people who meet activity guidelines in wealthier, industrialised countries like the UK fall under the semi-official public health category of 'weekend warriors'. Such people are largely immobile on weekdays, often with a sedentary job and commute, and try to make up for it with a burst of sport, or activities like gardening. The verdict on this activity pattern is slightly mixed, and yet again a lot of it comes from studies led or co-authored by the ubiquitous I-Min Lee.

An early attempt to look into this phenomenon, in 2004, found that for sixty-something weekend warriors at least, health gains were seen in people who did not have any risk factors, such as excess weight or a history of heart disease, but not those who did. In contrast, people who carried such a risk but were active throughout the week did experience benefits.[29]

But a more recent Lee-involved study from 2017, which followed more than 60,000 English and Scottish people aged forty or older, found that while regular activity brought greater benefits, weekend warriors were still around 30 per cent less likely to die over the average nine-year follow-up period than people who were inactive. Importantly, the study found there were even gains for weekend warriors who did not reach minimum activity guidelines. As the authors noted: 'Less frequent bouts of activity, which might be more easily fit into a busy lifestyle, offer considerable health benefits, even in the obese and those with major risk factors.'[30]

There is the message again, and it is one that cannot be stressed enough: there are remarkably few circumstances under which being physically active for even slightly longer, or a bit more vigorously, will not do you some good. This accumulation of knowledge about the health dividends of even relatively tiny amounts of exertion is, like Richard Mackenzie's examination of the cellular process of pre-diabetes, at the leading edge of inactivity research efforts. But as we will see in the next chapter, however numerous and varied the studies, they all ultimately originate from the same place: the remarkably little-known life and work of the extraordinary British scientist who first proved that everyday movement is good for us.

Next steps:

Try, if you can, to roughly tally how much activity you amass in an average week – how many minutes of moderate and/or vigorous movement. There are lots of useful web pages which give a full list of what activities count. You might be surprised how it all adds up, or you might realise you are, officially, inactive. And when you are walking, think about trying to do so briskly. Remember I-Min Lee's adage about being able to speak but not necessarily sing.

3

The Man Who Rediscovered Movement

In 1948, as Britain began to tentatively emerge from its post-war fug of austerity, a young doctor of formidable intellect and apparently limitless energy took on a job that might have been created especially for him. There, he quietly decided to see whether he could change the world.

This was Jerry Morris, a man whose amazing life story argu-ably merits an entire book of its own. Newly demobbed from service as an army doctor in India and Burma, Morris became director of the brand new Social Medicine Unit, a government-established body tasked with examining how health issues interact with people's real-life circumstances. Morris was a qui-etly fierce, endlessly tenacious advocate for the societal changes that would help people to stay healthier. He also knew from personal experience that someone's chances were greatly shaped by the background from which they came and the environment in which they lived.

It was Morris's stroke of genius to look into why the drivers of London's double-decker buses had significantly higher rates of heart attacks than their conductor colleagues, and to eventually conclude that the only real difference between the groups was that the former spent their working days sitting down, while the latter were constantly on their feet, tramping up and down flights of stairs. Everyday physical exertion had to be the answer. After making this breakthrough, Morris spent decades politely haranguing government ministers to take action over it. That he largely failed says much more about the sheer weight of political lassitude and indifference he faced than about his own energy and far-sightedness.

In fact, along with the slightly later but similarly influential work of Ralph Paffenbarger, a US pioneer of physical activity science who became a close collaborator and friend, Morris arguably did as much as any single academic to shape post-war thinking and knowledge. And yet, even in his own country Morris is barely known beyond specialist public health circles.

These days, the idea that staying physically active is generally good for you might seem so obvious that it is almost difficult to believe this was not always known. But Morris's landmark academic paper setting out his findings was only published in 1953, a few years after other researchers had connected smoking and cancer.

Even more extraordinarily from a modern viewpoint, the discovery was seen, at first, as significantly controversial. Part of this was the need to overturn decades of scientific orthodoxy, in particular the persistent if entirely ill-founded idea that significant physical effort was bad for the heart.

But also, the breakthrough came just as society-wide moves towards a more inactive world were really taking hold. Millions of people in Britain were gratefully enjoying the embrace of labour-saving household goods, and cars. They were, perhaps understandably, not so welcoming of the idea that the more gruelling, materially deprived period they had just been through might in some ways have been better for them. This arguably helped set the tone for subsequent decades of public and government inaction, something long apparent to Morris.

It is a paradox of Morris's discovery about movement and health that however contentious it was at the time, the idea would have seemed notably less surprising to practitioners a couple of millennia before. The history of medicine is littered with doctor-sages extolling the health benefits of regular exertion. Most famous was Hippocrates, the ancient Greek physician and founding figure of medicine, who 400 or so years before the birth of Jesus was pronouncing that 'food and exercise, while possessing opposite qualities, yet work together to produce health'. He was also the first medical practitioner recorded as prescribing movement as an individual treatment, writing that a patient with consumption should seek to walk regularly.

For centuries this was considered perfectly ordinary advice. 'Of all the causes which conspire to render the life of man short and miserable, none have greater influence than the want of proper exercise,' wrote William Buchan, the celebrated eighteenth-century Scottish doctor and author in his hugely popular book *Domestic Medicine*, a publishing phenomenon of the era which was translated into numerous languages.[1]

But as modern medicine emerged in the Victorian era, exertion began to be seen as almost a problem. Just under a century before Morris's discovery, another single-minded and now largely forgotten medic-campaigner, Edward Smith, who had already led a colourful life including a brief spell selling land to fellow Britons in Texas, investigated conditions at the evocatively named and long-closed Coldbath Fields Prison in London. There, inmates sentenced to hard labour were punished by spending several hours a day on a so-called treadwheel, where a long line of men would turn a huge, cylindrical wheel with steps on it by pushing down with their feet, as if ascending an endless flight of stairs.

Originally designed to pump water or mill grain, later tread-wheels, as in Coldbath Fields, just turned a fan, something the prisoners ruefully called 'grinding the wind'. Smith, who had a pioneering interest in measuring ventilatory volume – how much air someone breathes in and out – went to the prison with the assumption that such exertion would be inevitably bad for the prisoners' wellbeing, writing that it must 'induce disease and a premature death'. But when Smith actually examined them, he found, as you might expect, that their cardiovascular health seemed fine. What ailments they suffered, Smith discovered, were mainly caused by a diet that provided nowhere near the amount of nutrition needed for such a physical regime.[2]

By the time Morris and Paffenbarger were emerging, some tentative studies were being carried out into the long-term health impact of activity and exercise. But these seemed mainly based around the worry, popular since the Victorian era and tied inexorably to the in-built, snobbish assumption that a gentleman's chair-bound lifestyle must be the preferable one, that increasing one's heartbeat and raising a sweat was damaging for your health, not to mention a bit undignified.

In April 1939, with Morris a junior doctor in London and the slightly younger Paffenbarger about to start university, the prestigious *British Medical Journal* (*BMJ*) published a study titled *The Longevity of Oarsmen*, which examined the lifespans of those who had crewed the Oxford and Cambridge rowing boats in the celebrated annual inter-university race between 1829 and 1929.

Led by the floridly named Sir Percival Horton-Smith Hartley from St Bart's Hospital in London, it took with complete seriousness the notion that vigorous exercise could be dangerous.

The authors approvingly cited the opinion of one medical expert that such a boat race was 'a national folly', as well as the view expressed by one early participant that 'no man in a racing-boat could expect to live to the age of 30'.

As it transpired, Horton-Smith Hartley's research found that those who had taken part in the race actually seemed to live longer than average. However, he carefully caveated this finding with warnings that the sample size was small, and that the comparison death rates came from the everyday population, rather than the oarsmen's social and educational peers.[3]

Even more striking in retrospect is another *BMJ* study, also centring on the much-scrutinised lifespans of elite academic alumni. Carried out by Sir Alan Rook, the senior health officer at Cambridge University, it again considered the potential perils of vigorous exercise. Strikingly, it was published in April 1954 – five months after Morris's research paper on London bus workers.

As was still the received wisdom, Rook fretted mainly about the impact of exercise on the heart, noting this was 'usually regarded as bearing the chief strain of athletic activities'. While it was now generally believed that exercise caused no immediate ill-effect on a normal heart, he wrote, whether or not it might bring longer-term cardiac damage is 'the part of the problem that has never been answered satisfactorily'.

Using the death records of thirty years of Cambridge alumni, the study compared a cohort of students who had taken part in university sports against a control group, as well as an 'intellectual group' and a 'random group'. A curious amalgam of scientific rigour and highly set social assumptions, the paper talks breezily of 'weaklings' being weeded out by around the age of forty, and notes in passing that an alarmingly high proportion of Cambridge intellectuals from the era ended up killing themselves. But again, in the end it managed to uncover no evidence that the reckless sportsmen died any younger on average than their peers.[4]

The quiet radical

It was into this curious post-war intellectual environment that Jerry Morris arrived. The son of immigrant parents who had fled pogroms in what is now Belarus, he had emerged from an upbringing notably limited in material wealth but rich in love, culture and omnivorous intellectual curiosity.

Morris was, according to those who knew and worked with him, a seemingly mild but iron-willed force of nature; a lifelong socialist who happily and mischievously described himself as 'a radical – a do-gooder'; someone who thought nothing of personally telephoning ministers to lambast them about policy failures; but who also quietly helped along the careers of junior colleagues, often without their knowledge.

According to a family history compiled by a contemporary example of Morris's seemingly endless list of eclectic and over-achieving relatives (Joshua Plaut, who combines a role as a rabbi in New York City with being a photographer and the author of books including *A Kosher Christmas: 'Tis the Season to be Jewish*), Morris's parents came to the UK in 1909, fleeing increased anti-semitism in the then-Russian city of Novogrudok.[5]

Once arrived, Natke Lezerovsky and Chaya Yoselovsky, in their early twenties and recently married, become Nathan and Annie Morris, supposedly adopting the surname of the friendly captain of the boat that carried them to Liverpool. They tried their luck in Glasgow, and flourished. By 1912, Nathan was headmaster of a Hebrew school in the city, later going on to take a master's degree in literature at Glasgow University. According to one version of the family story, after finishing the degree

Nathan then declared, to his wife's dismay, that an educated man must also know about music, and spent two further years studying that.

In a fascinating video interview from 1986,[6] when Jerry Morris had already been officially retired for more than a decade but was still arriving daily at his office in the London School of Hygiene and Tropical Medicine, he described, in an accent still thick with his Glasgow roots, how he and his two younger brothers were 'brought up on a mixture of the Old Testament and the Independent Labour Party', a firebrand socialist grouping which had emerged in Scotland a decade or so before his birth. Morris explained: 'It has given me a rather simple view of life. I mean, I've got less problems with what's right and what's wrong than other people.'

Morris and his two brothers – who became a trade union leader and a paediatrician – had all grown up in a tiny Glasgow house of two bedrooms and a kitchen. 'We were next door to a slum street,' Morris recalled in an interview from 2009. 'I still remember the screaming women on Friday night and Saturday night, when they were beaten by their drunk husbands. As you can imagine, I have a contact with social inequalities and with poverty that most of my colleagues only know from the literature.'[7] While he played down the deprivation the family faced personally, it was an upbringing still challenging enough to leave Morris with lifelong traces of rickets, the childhood bone weakness condition so strongly associated with poverty.

Another legacy was adherence to a personal form of socialism, the beginnings of which saw Morris volunteer to campaign for a local Labour MP in Glasgow, being turned away because he was, at the time, aged only twelve. This childhood gave him not only a very personal insight into the many problems of deprivation, but also a grounding in what for him was the other side of the health equation: being physically active. His hugely energetic father, Morris recalled, would take him and his brothers for a four-mile walk across Glasgow once a week as children. If they managed the route inside an hour, the boys would be rewarded with an ice cream. Walk the distance in a notably shorter time and the prize was upgraded to a choc-ice.

Morris had wanted from childhood to become a doctor, but initially studied a combination of arts and medicine at Glasgow University at the urging of his polymath father, who 'thought that doctors were a very uneducated lot'. After the family relocated to London, Morris continued his training at University College Hospital, where his combined proclivities for quiet determination and being in the right place at the right time saw him work under first the famous cardiologist Thomas Lewis and then another celebrated doctor, Frederic Poynton. Poynton was an expert in rheumatic fever, the inflammatory disease which can badly damage hearts, particularly in children. Now almost unknown in the developed world, in the London of the 1930s it remained common. In his 1986 interview, Morris remembered the shock of being told by a senior doctor that his very first patient, an eight-year-old boy with heart valves damaged from rheumatic fever, would most likely live only a few more months. 'It took me days to get over that,' Morris recalled.[8] The impact was all the greater when Poynton mentioned that in many years treating private patients in London's upmarket Harley Street, and at the elite Eton school, he had never seen a single case of rheumatic heart disease. This was entirely a disease of poverty.

Morris's increasing belief that combating illness was a matter of changing living conditions became even stronger when he met Richard Titmuss, a celebrated researcher who more or less single-handedly established the academic discipline of social policy, which examines how governments can tackle issues such as education and health. Titmuss is another extraordinary character whose life and achievements are not as well known as they could be, particularly given his billing as one of the intellectual founders of the UK's welfare state. The son of a Bedfordshire farmer, Titmuss left school at fourteen and found work as an insurance clerk. Hugely intelligent and often self-taught, and with a deep knowledge of statistics and demographics from his day job, he began writing books, including one on regional differences in public health.

Morris read this and physically tracked down Titmuss in his London insurance office after – as he put it years later – 'deciding, well, this is a man I must know'.[9] The pair became close friends and began working on projects in what they termed 'medicine in the matrix of society', the emerging discipline that became known as social medicine.

Their work, crucial in shaping Morris's later ideas, continued even after Morris was sent abroad during the war with the Royal Army Medical Corps, the military censors allowing their endless stream of letters to pass unamended. 'They must have had a meeting at a high level and decided to leave these screwballs alone,' said Morris. 'There was no danger of secret information being conveyed in these statistics on death rates in the county boroughs of England and Wales or whatever it was we were writing on.'[10]

From 1942 to 1944 Morris and Titmuss published three papers now seen as the origins of social medicine, covering conditions closely linked with poverty and lifestyle – juvenile rheumatism, peptic ulcers and rheumatic heart disease. The latter, which had so cursed the brief life of Morris's first patient, was described by the duo as a 'social disease', something they demonstrated in part by correlating its incidence against levels of unemployment.

The papers attracted attention, and took Morris towards the

role that would define his career, and change public health forever. In 1948, the 38-year-old Morris was made head of the Social Medicine Unit. He kept it until his official retirement almost three decades later, although in fact he never actually stopped working until weeks before his death.

A grandly titled enterprise with humble beginnings – it started in a single portacabin in the grounds of a London hospital – the Social Medicine Unit was charged with investigating population-wide health trends and examining what might be causing them. This is now treated as routine in public health, but during the years following the Second World War was a pioneering adjunct to the conventional care which was now being provided free to everyone for the first time via the brand new National Health Service.

In an interview many years later Morris explained his thinking in 1948: 'Starting the unit, I asked myself, what is the great presenting problem?'[11] Morris's answer was simple: coronary heart disease. The condition, most dramatically and terrifyingly manifested in people suffering sudden and fatal heart attacks, had long been understood from a basic physiological perspective, but there had been remarkably little curiosity as to what factors triggered it. Some concern had been expressed following the war about an increase in the incidence of heart attacks, but there was little study as to the extent of the problem, let alone contributory causes, beyond some tentative guesses about workplace stress or a possible link to the bitumen being used to resurface roads amid peacetime rebuilding efforts.

Morris began his work with the sort of thorough if gloomy endeavour familiar to many who specialise in social medicine and epidemiology: he studied lots and lots of mortality records. Morris ploughed through files detailing all those who had died from heart-related ailments at the London Hospital in the East

End of the city between 1907 and 1949. After what he later described as 'interminable hours with post-mortem folios',[12] he discovered two things: firstly that the incidence of heart disease was, indeed, rising from a previously low base; and also that it was more prevalent in men than in women. 'It appeared that this ancient disease had been mutating from relative obscurity into the modern epidemic of heart attack,' he wrote in 2009.[13]

The next step saw Morris and his team assess coronary heart disease rates across large cohorts of people, exclusively men, who worked in differing jobs in a variety of sectors, among them postal staff, civil servants and London Transport workers. It was the latter group who provided his team with their initial breakthrough.

Amid the paternalistic culture of the era there was masses of data already available about such people from their employers, not just sickness rates and statistics for those who became ill or died from heart disease, but details on social background and work practices, even in some cases the waistband sizes of the uniform trousers issued to them.

Morris and his colleagues pored over figures for 31,000 London Transport staff working on buses, trams and the Underground. One anomaly soon emerged: bus conductors had about half the rates of heart disease of their colleagues who drove the vehicles. Their backgrounds and other biographical details tended to be similar, so it must be the jobs which had the impact. But how?

In the 1986 interview, Morris said he initially looked back to his cardiology teachings under Thomas Lewis, much of which would have been familiar to a Victorian doctor, and concluded it was most likely down to differing levels of work stress. The research team spent many hours observing both occupations in action, but started to question this hypothesis. 'Eventually we managed to articulate between us that both of these jobs were stressful,' Morris said. 'But what was interesting about this was, [the researchers] said if they had to pick one of these jobs as being the more stressful they would say it was the conductor, and for why, because the conductor had to deal with people whereas the driver only had to deal with traffic.'[14] Body weight was also considered, thanks to the London Transport records on trouser sizes. But although the bus drivers tended to be fatter on average, conductors with a certain body type still suffered fewer sudden cardiac deaths than the equivalent-shaped drivers.

However, the long observations had uncovered another difference. 'The drivers were prototypically sedentary and the conductors were unavoidably active.' Morris recounted. 'We spent many hours sitting on the buses watching the number of stairs they climbed.'[15] It turned out that in an average working day, conductors climbed and descended between 500 and 750 steps.

The decision was made. 'In the face of much collegial scepticism, we chose to focus on physical activity,' Morris wrote in 2009, adding that 'British cardiology was quite uninterested in what we were doing.'[16] Morris was, of course, correct in this hypothesis, which was backed up by the data. However, desperate to be certain he was correct, he and his team spent three further years checking their conclusion and gathering more evidence.

'Nowadays we'd have rushed this into print overnight,' Morris remarked to a fellow academic many years later. 'In fact we decided to test it every way we could before publishing.'[17] This testing came in two variants. Firstly, Morris called in other academics to scrutinise the findings. 'We brought in outside people with no blood in their veins, no interest, to destroy it,' he recalled.[18] But they could find no error. Then, finally, evidence started to arrive from the other occupational studies set up by the team. In what Morris later called 'one of the tensest moments of my professional life',[19] he received data about postal workers, which showed that postmen who delivered mail by bike or on foot also had roughly half the incidence of heart disease as their inactive colleagues, the clerks and counter staff.

Finally convinced his hypothesis was sound, Morris submitted the article to leading medical journal *The Lancet*, where it appeared in issue 6795, on 28 November 1953, under the sober and succinct title, *Coronary Heart Disease and Physical Activity of Work*.

As part of my research into the family history, I visit Tamara Lucas, whose father was Morris's cousin and grew up alongside him in Glasgow. By coincidence, Lucas works for Elsevier, the publishing giant whose titles include *The Lancet*. We meet at its central London office, where she leads me to the magazine's archive, a small room with floor-to-ceiling shelves filled with original copies, many pages featuring the authors' handwritten corrections and annotations.

She pulls down from the shelves the bound volume containing the relevant magazine issue.

Morris's study, with his name one of five academics at the top, begins with the modest aspiration that it hopes to 'gain some knowledge of coronary heart disease as a problem in public health'. Over five densely typed pages, embellished with tables and hand-drawn graphs, the authors explain how the finding that active bus conductors had lower rates of heart disease than drivers was then backed by observations of postal workers, including civil service postal staff. It concludes: 'We felt that the main interest of these findings in postal workers and civil servants lies in the support they provide for the idea suggested by the observation of the transport workers – that physical activity at work is important in relation to the coronary heart disease of middle-aged men.'

The article prompted, as Morris put it more than half a century later, a wave of interest 'that I had no idea how to handle'. A good proportion of this was hostile. Could a desk-bound professional life – the norm for millions of middle- and upper-class men, and a major aspiration for those who still laboured for a living – really be to blame for the new epidemic of heart attacks?

It can be difficult from a modern perspective to appreciate how radical Morris's conclusions were. I-Min Lee, the Harvard epidemiology professor we met in the last chapter, is generally considered the successor to Morris and Paffenbarger. She stresses how much of a risk Morris was taking with his hypothesis: 'He did this at a time when nobody believed activity was important,' she says. 'People thought this was a crazy thing he was doing.'[20]

But for the critics there was one problem: the evidence kept on arriving. Morris and his team expanded their observations to non-work activity, tracking the health of thousands of relatively senior civil servants, none of whom were physical in their jobs. Among this group, he found, men who undertook reasonably vigorous exercise, for example swimming, cycling or brisk walking, had lower rates of heart attacks than their more sedentary peers.

Morris was also now not alone in his efforts, with researchers in various countries starting to build on his work. In 1961, a pair of US-based academics, Hans Kraus and Wilhelm Raab, published the first book detailing the health consequences of a world where, as they put it, physical exertion 'has been taken over, step-by-step, by labour-saving devices'. The book, *Hypokinetic Disease: Diseases Produced by Lack of Exercise*, expanded its list of ailments caused by inactivity beyond heart disease, also citing metabolic disorders and mental health.[21]

The fate of freshmen

But it was another US academic who was to become Morris's key ally, as well as a close friend, and a researcher whose achievements in the field would be seen as perhaps equal: Ralph Paffenbarger. Known universally to colleagues as Paff, he had a notably more conventional background than Morris, as the son of a faculty member from Ohio State University. Graduating as a doctor during the Second World War before moving into epidemiology, Paffenbarger began by researching the transmission of polio for the US Public Health Service, a branch of the military.

His primary contribution, when he started to examine the impact of active lifestyles, was to support Morris's initial findings with far larger, long-term studies. Paffenbarger also helped spark the exercise boom that swept America in the 1970s, albeit more or less by accident.

Paffenbarger began with a study of longshoremen, or dock workers, in San Francisco. In total 3,263 men who had varying levels of physical activity in their work, and now largely extinct job titles such as shoveller, holdman, sugarman, winchdriver, cooper and walking boss, were examined for other differences such as weight, blood pressure and whether or not they smoked. In a pioneering example of the longitudinal studies which now form the bedrock of much of epidemiology, Paffenbarger and his team returned sixteen years later, by which time 888 of the men had died, 291 from heart attacks. The eventual 1970 paper found that after accounting for other lifestyle and health factors, those with the least active jobs suffered coronary heart deaths a third higher than those in strenuous roles such as cargo handling – who, the study found, expended an average of 925 more calories per eight-hour shift.[22]

Paffenbarger's major achievement was the subsequent College

Alumni Health Study, a vast linear record of physical activity and associated health, begun in 1960 and initially focusing on Harvard. Covering those who entered college between 1916 and 1950 – again all men – it was helped enormously by the painstaking record keeping maintained by the elite university. Until late in the 1950s, Harvard had required all newly arrived freshmen to take a medical examination, giving an initial set of data Paffenbarger could compare with his own results. Harvard also kept a close eye on its ex-students, with the alumni office receiving a weekly 'death list'.

For the former students still living, Paffenbarger compiled what he called a physical activity index, getting them to fill in questionnaires on exertion, such as how many flights of stairs they tended to climb, and how far they walked, as well as details on 'light sports', such as golf, and 'strenuous sports', such as basketball and running. This was then compared to death rates and levels of illness in what Paffenbarger later called 'a natural history of ways of life and disease in America'.

The eventual 1978 research paper, which charted 16,936 male Harvard alumni aged between thirty-five and seventy-four, 572 of whom had suffered heart attacks, found that those who described low levels of activity had a 64 per cent higher risk of heart attack than those who were more consistently physical, with strenuous exercise bringing the most benefits. It also discovered that being a college athlete offered no apparent protection from heart attack unless levels of physical activity were maintained.[23]

The study was concluded with a report in 1986, which definitively concluded that whether or not people had other risk factors such as smoking, obesity or psychological trauma, 'alumni mortality rates were significantly lower among the physically active'.[24]

Paffenbarger's work followed on from Morris's breakthrough, proving beyond any doubt how important physical activity is for continued health, and inspiring generations of new researchers to discover other benefits which come from such a life. One of these was I-Min Lee, whose work at Harvard includes stewardship of the seemingly never-ending college alumni project, as well as a parallel exercise chronicling the lives of nearly 40,000 middle-aged and older women.[25]

Lee says Paffenbarger's legacy is immense. 'Now we know that one of the best things you can do for your health is be physically active,' she tells me. 'Ralph Paffenbarger used to say that anything that gets worse as you grow older gets better when you exercise. It's incredibly true – not only do we now know that physical activity reduces our risk of a whole bunch of chronic diseases, helps us live longer, but it also improves our quality of life.'[26]

Practising what they preached

One of Paffenbarger's early and notable findings was that physical activity seems to boost a person's health outcomes even if they take it up for the first time in middle age. This was to have particular resonance for the then largely desk-bound scientist, whose immediate family included several men who had died from heart attacks in their fifties.

At the age of forty-five, in 1967, Paffenbarger decided to put his ideas to the test and take up jogging. Lee recalls him saying later that he was prompted to do this because his oldest child was newly in college and was having a difficult time. Paffenbarger wanted 'to sort of show his son that if you put your mind to it, you can get through anything difficult. So he decided to run a marathon,' Lee says.

Early efforts were unpromising. 'It was terrible,' Paffenbarger said in a 1996 interview. 'I was exhausted by the end of the block. I was delighted to be behind the junior high school, where no one could see me.'[27] But he persisted: 'By the second week, I was hooked.' Notably, Paffenbarger also hailed the mental effects as a reason for his epiphany: 'I found it invigorating. I could consider my thoughts and conflicts, I could prepare letters, ponder problems, prepare talks.'[28]

According to Lee, Paffenbarger still didn't immediately buy proper running footwear, and took part in his first Boston Marathon later that year wearing boating shoes, finishing just over five hours later with several toenails covered in blood from the chafing. But he turned out to be a natural athlete, and within four years he was running the distance in less than two hours forty-five minutes. He went on to complete about 150 marathons.

By the time Paffenbarger was a committed runner, the first wider wave of joggers was emerging across America, many inspired by Ken Cooper, a doctor and air force colonel who in 1968 published a bestselling book called *Aerobics*,[29] then a new term to most, setting out the importance of exercise to long-term health. But it is worth noting that when Cooper began his advocacy it was based entirely on personal belief. In a tribute in *Runner's World* magazine after Paffenbarger's death in 2007, the US runner-turned-writer Amby Burfoot said Cooper admitted he had at first made no more than 'an educated guess' that jogging was actually good for people. 'As he once told me, he had no idea if all the joggers he created might keel over and die during their workouts,' Burfoot wrote of Cooper. 'Paff proved that Cooper was right.'

It is a curiosity of Paffenbarger's influence that while his work was devoted to studying the benefits of everyday movement, his extracurricular life as a committed runner meant it was also adopted by the minority who take part in such sports. His work, Burfoot said, 'stands as the very foundation of the exercise and fitness movement we all believe in so strongly'. Burfoot added: 'Paff was the guy who got things started. He was the pioneer.'[30]

Morris, by contrast, would never have seen himself as an 'athlete', just someone who saw the benefit in always being physically active, including the habit instilled by his father of setting off on brisk walks whenever feasible. Liam Donaldson, who went on to become England's chief medical officer, the most senior adviser to government on health matters, recalls that as a junior lecturer at Leicester University he was sent out in a car to collect Morris from the local station and drive him to deliver a talk. But on learning the distance was only one and a half miles Morris insisted they walk, and spent the trek grilling the young academic on the useful public health people he should know in the city.[31]

An avid reader of other health research, Morris had noticed the findings in the 1950s of Richard Doll, another pioneering epidemiologist, into the link between smoking and lung cancer, and immediately gave up his cigarette habit. Later he began jogging, though in a manner which would seem unrecognisable to Paffenbarger, let alone to Ken Cooper. 'I was the first person to run on Hampstead Heath, in the 1960s,' he said in 2009. 'Every Sunday morning, if the weather was at all possible, I took off my coat, and my little boy carried my coat, I took off my jacket, and my little girl carried my jacket, and I ran for twenty minutes. People thought I was bananas.'[32]

He was also a keen swimmer, taking any opportunity that arose. Mervyn Hillsdon, an Exeter University epidemiologist who collaborated with Morris on several of his later studies, recalls attending an academic event in the 1980s: 'I was waiting for a lift to go back up to my room at a conference. He was coming down, dressed in his swimming hat, goggles and a robe, on his way to the pool. That's how we first met.'

Morris was by then in his mid-seventies, and continued swimming well into his nineties. He only stopped, Hillsdon says, because the aftermath of a broken hip made his walking uneven and he was 'a bit nervous around the edge of the pool in case he fell'. Morris himself said he gave up because he was embarrassed by people rushing to help him when he got out of the water. Even afterwards he would still walk on Hampstead Heath and trek up the stairs to his office. 'He really believed that on every day of his life he should take some exercise,' Hillsdon said.[33]

According to Lee, Morris can perhaps best be seen as 'more of the everyman for physical activity', as opposed to the marathon-running Paffenbarger. 'He walked, he swam, and he swam into his nineties. So he did the kind of things that people can do when they get old. Ralph Paffenbarger is a bit of an anomaly. I think it might be a bit harder to identify with him. He turned out to be genetically very good in terms of exercise. But, interestingly, I don't think he'd have known it if he hadn't taken it up.'[34]

Both regimes clearly worked. Paffenbarger remained trim and energetic to the end of his life, while Morris appeared to barely slow down even in very old age. 'Jerry Morris is one of those lucky few in whom the ageing process starts normally, then admits defeat and gives up,' began a *BMJ* tribute to him on his ninetieth birthday.[35]

Morris never wavered in either his habits or his advocacy of them to others. 'It's the only way in which I feel entitled, as an old buffer, to give advice to people,' he said shortly before his death. 'I'm constantly being asked: "Your long life, what would you advise?" and so forth. To start telling other people what to do, I'm very reluctant. Except on exercise, where to a large extent I feel it's what I've done myself that's contributed to longevity.'[36]

It marches together with the human condition

While they worked on opposite sides of an ocean, and never directly collaborated on any studies, the ties between these two figures who pioneered the discovery behind this book remained close, and the wider academic community recognised the connection in their achievements. Perhaps the ultimate sign of this influence came in 1996, when, at the Atlanta Summer Olympics, Paffenbarger and Morris were jointly awarded gold medals for sports science by the International Olympic Committee, the first time such a prize had been given.

Paffenbarger eventually died from complications connected to heart disease aged eighty-four, having reputedly been not just delighted but surprised to outstrip his family history of early male deaths.

Lee says that Morris and Paffenbarger used to speak by phone every week, and when the latter died, she stepped in: 'They were very good friends. When Paff died I felt like I had almost inherited a relative from him, and I should continue calling Jerry. We didn't manage it as often, but I'd call to see what he was up to.'

In legacy, however, the two researchers can be seen as slightly different. Paffenbarger's direct influence is arguably more connected to his academic peers, as the scientist who pioneered the mass-scale, years-long population studies which are the foundation of modern public health research. Aside from further proving Morris's ideas about physical activity, Paffenbarger's work expanded the list of conditions affected by activity, such as strokes, and introduced a series of ideas which remain the inspiration for current studies, for example the impact of exercise on people of different weight types.

In a tribute published soon after Paffenbarger died, Lee and some colleagues noted the statistics which highlight his influence. Most academic papers are never cited by any other studies, she wrote, and even those which are mentioned generally gather fewer than ten citations. Those with 50 are viewed as 'classics'. Over his long career, Lee noted, Paffenbarger published 187 research papers, which had by then amassed more than 20,000 citations, and were gaining at least another 1,000 every year.[37]

Much as with their respective sporting efforts, Morris could perhaps be seen as more of a real-world academic, closely connected to the ways in which his ideas affect people in their everyday lives, sometimes to an almost unlikely degree of detail.

He was intimately aware of how these social factors could change. While his 1930s patients faced conditions like rheumatic heart disease due to a lack of available medical care, as the decades went on, poverty affected people's health in different ways. When more than fifty years later Morris contributed to government work on deciding a new minimum wage, he ordered officials to price in the cost of a decent pair of walking shoes, as well as the cost of tea and biscuits a certain number of times a week, recognising that mobility and sociability are both significant factors in good health outcomes.[38]

Morris completely understood that public health is shaped by the physical and cultural environment. He endlessly lobbied for more sports facilities – 'Swimming means there must be pools,' he said[39] – as well as routes for safe cycling and convenient walking. He was hugely interested in how his field was dealt with in the media. 'Jerry is the only person who tells me I ought to watch more television, not less,' remarked Michael Marmot, one of the most eminent current epidemiologists, who led a landmark 2010 study into UK health inequalities.[40]

This broad approach was fed by an omnivorous attitude to knowledge typical of the son of the much-educated Nathan Morris. Tamara Lucas recalls that when, as an anthropology student, she would visit him, he would generally take her on a long walk to a swimming pool. On the way Morris would quiz her endlessly about her subject. 'He knew about everything,' she says. 'He was one of those very erudite people. I can't imagine what I would have been studying that he wouldn't have been interested in.'[41] Hillsdon notes that Morris's small social medicine department included not just epidemiologists but a series of other disciplines, for example physiologists and historians: 'He loved spending time with people who came at the same topic that he was interested in from a completely different methodological approach. It's something he told me all the time – always have conversations with a really broad range of disciplines and specialists, because otherwise there's a risk of becoming too narrow in your thinking.'

This external-facing view of his science saw Morris not just produce the raw evidence for the benefits of more widespread physical activity, but spend increasing amounts of time trying to persuade people to act on it. According to Hillsdon, Morris regularly penned handwritten letters to government ministers and others in positions of influence to warn them about the consequences for public health if they did not take action. Hillsdon adds: 'If they simply ignored him he'd get on the phone and say, "I'm surprised you didn't have the courtesy to acknowledge receipt of my letter. I'm wondering whether that meant it didn't arrive?"'[42]

Morris was the lead researcher in one of the first official reports to fully highlight how inactive the UK population had become. The National Fitness Survey carried out exhaustive interviews and fitness tests with thousands of people during 1990, with the subsequent report highlighting not only the number of Britons unable to carry out even fairly basic physical tasks, but a worrying lack of awareness among many people about their own lack of fitness.

The study found that over two thirds of women and nearly a third of men would find it difficult to maintain an average-speed walk (at 3mph) up a slight gradient. Among older people, those aged fifty-five to seventy-four, more than half of women and almost a third of men would struggle to do this even on level ground, having to slow or stop after about ten minutes. In practical movement terms, this amounted to having a disability.[43]

Throughout his life Morris worked to produce more such research – in later years often omitting his age from grant applications to boost the chances of success – and badgered successive generations of government ministers and chief medical officers. But even he could not stem the tide. This was, Hillsdon says, a source of endless frustration: 'It used to drive him nuts. Jerry always said, "My great failure has been that I never really influenced policymakers, and they never really took physical activity seriously enough." It wasn't about his science – it was about his ability to influence people who could change policy as a result of the science.' In the interview from 2009, Morris was more blunt: 'Just imagine what historians in the future are going to say about the way we've allowed this epidemic of childhood obesity. "Disgrace" is a sort of mild word.'[44]

Even as the importance of physical activity for health becomes ever-more prominent, the two men who did most to prove the link remain generally unknown outside academic circles. When they died, Morris and Paffenbarger received brief if glowing obituaries in a handful of newspapers, but if you mention either to someone outside a relatively limited field of public health or associated fields, you're likely to get a blank look.

'Jerry was an extremely humble man and didn't like to give his studies big titles to increase their profile,' says Hillsdon. 'He was more concerned with the quality of the science than anything else.' Tamara Lucas, whose father grew up alongside Morris in their large, bustling, ever-enquiring extended family in the now barely recognisable world of pre-war Glasgow, agrees: 'Jerry was very modest. He was never pushy or self-promoting. I never heard him boast about what he did. But his influence is extraordinary – it's a shame that he's not as acknowledged as he could be.'

Among the many discoveries built on his work are studies which have shown how remaining physically active is a key factor in warding off mental decline. Again, Morris's life provides a resonant example. Family and colleagues say that Morris never seemed to slow down mentally. In October 2009 he eventually died, aged ninety-nine and a half. 'He always insisted on adding the half,' recalled his daughter, Julie.[45] He had spent his last days in a London hospital, severely weakened by pneumonia and kidney failure. But even here Morris remained eager to exchange ideas. Through his oxygen mask he endlessly quizzed staff and fellow patients on what they thought about a then-ongoing strike by postal workers, and a recent rise in prominence for the far-right British National Party. At Morris's funeral his son, David, had said he never expected the moment to come, as his father had seemingly found the secret of, if not eternal existence, then one that seemed to be prolonged for the foreseeable future.[46]

Morris's life and research contain lessons which could bring greater longevity, not to mention hugely improved quality of life, to millions of other people around the world. That governments have not as yet heeded this message is in no way the responsibility of Morris, arguably one of the most prodigious, influential and yet relatively little-celebrated figures of the past century.

Next steps:

Jerry Morris was very much not an athlete. But he was always very active. Try some of his methods, perhaps even walking a mile and a half from a train station, rather than driving, or at least up the stairs when you can. If you have younger children, you could even test out the ice cream–based bribes for particularly long and brisk walks.

4

The Tidal Wave: How Inactivity is Bankrupting Governments

Interviewing a doctor inside the emergency department of a busy inner-city hospital is rarely easy, but Martin Whyte is enjoying what is – by his standards, if that of few others – a fairly relaxed morning at the office. He has just helped examine the newest patient to reach King's College Hospital, a clearly very weak man in his eighties, with dementia, brought in from a care home. A series of other recent arrivals groan or lie silent behind curtain screens. But almost half the beds are empty, a rare sight at the usually frantic south London teaching hospital. Whyte thus has a brief moment to interrupt his chat with a junior doctor to answer the question I posed about five minutes earlier: what proportion of patients he sees are admitted due to conditions where inactive living can be identified as a factor?

Whyte pauses some more to look around the long, starkly lit, rectangular space, as other staff dart between cubicles or rapidly type notes into portable computer terminals set atop wheeled stands. 'That is basically my job,' he says eventually. 'It's people who are sedentary. Of course, it's not everyone, but it's a lot. And it's a big range of conditions: diabetes, heart disease, arthritis, dementia. You name it.'[1]

Whyte's observation is based on years of first-hand, expert experience, but there is an extent to which he is merely stating the obvious. As the statistics show, in the UK, or indeed in many dozens of other countries, if you are a professional of more or less any sort who deals with the adult public then a relatively high proportion of the people you encounter will live dangerously sedentary lives. The difference for Whyte and his colleagues, of course, is that they witness the moments when these years of inaction manifest themselves on someone's health, often in sudden and frightening ways.

This is, as we shall see, a phenomenon which, when repeated across populations, threatens to make universal medical systems like those in the UK increasingly unviable, and similarly threatens state care for older people. Make no mistake: just about every expert and policymaker agrees that without significant policy changes the only debate is about when all this will happen, not if.

During my day at King's examining this front line – this is before coronavirus erupts – I have two expert guides. The first is Whyte, a trim, cheery man in rolled-up sleeves and a waistcoat, who bounds along endless corridors and down several stairwells from his cramped office to the emergency department where, as a consultant, a senior doctor, he works with the accident and emergency team and their rapidly filling allocation of beds. Later I trail after Phil Kelly, another consultant. He is taller, even more lean, and strides back to his office from a ward round at such a pace I have to break into a trot to keep up. Both cheerily note the paradox that having a job tending to the chronically immobile seems to involve ceaseless walking. 'I'll be exhausted by the time I finish tonight, but at least I won't have to worry about being inactive,' Whyte grins.

Whyte and Kelly are both consultants in general medicine, that is to say the mass of everyday complaints not cordoned off by more specialist areas. Some of the patients they see will end up being moved to other departments, but they and their teams are the first point of contact, and oversee the broadest mass of hospital admissions. A significant percentage of their clientele arrive due to ailments closely associated with inactive lives, and the attendant, if separate, public health scourge of obesity. This could involve heart disease, difficulties in breathing, complications around arthritis, or, Whyte's particular focus, the rising tide of type 2 diabetes. If this wasn't alarming enough, more and more of their patients are presenting themselves with several of these lifestyle-induced conditions, and are likely to live with them for ever-longer periods.

Whyte introduces me to two medical terms which sum up this worrying new trend – co-morbidity and polypharmacy. The first describes patients with this series of interlinked, chronic medical issues. Co-morbidity, Whyte notes, used to be the preserve of older people. 'You're seeing that now at a much younger age – middle age rather than old age,' Whyte says. 'They'll have the burdens of diabetes, heart disease, stroke, osteoarthritis, blood clots – and around ten to fifteen years earlier than used to be the case, because of the impact of inactivity and weight. And one thing often begets another.'

Polypharmacy is simply what follows for such people: an indefinite future of permanent, multiple medications, a bind for them and a desperate financial strain for the health service. 'The minute someone's told they've got diabetes, they're on about five drugs,' Whyte says. 'It's the same with heart disease. And that's an expense. It's a tidal wave that's engulfing the NHS.'

We are just seventy years from the creation of the NHS, one of the world's earliest universal healthcare systems. The first year of the service, 1948, saw a health budget of about £370 million, or around £10.5 billion at modern prices.[2] Seven decades later, with a population that has grown only by about 25 per cent, the sum has swollen to £114 billion.[3] How did we get to a point where even this isn't enough?

Mortality and morbidity

As we saw in Chapter 2, the best estimates of the global death toll from illness linked to inactive living put it at beyond 5 million people a year, possibly significantly more. It forms part of a wider shift in healthcare focus from infectious viral and bacterial illnesses and onto so-called non-communicable diseases, or NCDs, which are often linked to lifestyle or environment. To an extent, this focus has shifted back with the sudden arrival of coronavirus. But even here NCDs play a key role, given an emerging link between conditions like diabetes and high blood pressure and poor coronavirus outcomes.

Academics gauge the impact of NCDs using a tool called Burden of Disease, which simply multiplies the risk an ailment poses to an individual by the extent of its spread. This system has been used to devise what public health officials call the 'four by four' threat – a list of the four most damaging NCDs around the world, and the four primary risk factors behind them. The ailments are much as you would expect: cardiovascular diseases, cancer, chronic respiratory diseases, and diabetes. As for the risk factors, these are equally predictable: tobacco, alcohol, obesity and inactivity.

Given the extent of inactivity and the amount of ill-health it causes, what overall impact does all this have on health services? The brief answer is: an extremely significant one. As well as risking the financial sustainability of many health and care systems, there are even worries for the future integrity of entire national economies.

There is a vital if counterintuitive point to make here. A significant element of these interlocked crises comes not from a failing but from a success – how good modern health services are at keeping people alive. Callous as it might sound, in financial terms the issue is less the sheer number of people who die, rather the millions who spend years or decades facing increasingly poor health, while often requiring regular medical check-ups and an arsenal of drugs.

It all comes down to the difference between mortality – people who die – and morbidity, a ubiquitous term in public health circles which simply describes the independence, good health and quality of life, or otherwise, of those who remain alive. This latter term gives its name to co-morbidity, the interconnected series of long-term medical conditions in individual patients which occupies so much of Martin Whyte's professional life at King's. And morbidity, particularly co-morbidity, is a lot more expensive than mortality.

The brutal truth is that dead people don't cost the taxpayer much. I once asked a professor of epidemiology to privately outline what would be the ideal lifespan of a citizen purely from the point of view of government economic efficiency. He replied: someone who works diligently and pays taxes their entire adult life, and on the day of their retirement, collapses and dies instantly from a massive heart attack (ideally, he added, with a demise so instantaneous and obvious that the bereaved family don't even bother to call an ambulance).

This is actually not so far from what used to be the case for many people only a few decades ago. As recently as 1961, UK male life expectancy was only sixty-eight,[4] giving the average man around three years in which to kick back and claim the state pension before he was no longer a drain on the public purse. The more basic medical care of the era, plus factors like a male smoking rate of about 70 per cent,[5] meant many people died fairly rapidly, without a prolonged period of illness or decrepitude. Heart attacks were particularly relevant here. The current UK death rate from cardiovascular disease per head of population is less than a third of what it was in 1961.[6]

It's worth stressing the perhaps obvious point that people living longer lives is, of course, a good thing. The only issue is the fact that so many millions experience longer periods of poor health, with this extension happening on both sides of the timeline – as well as living longer, people increasingly develop chronic conditions at an earlier age.

The UK is a prime example of this phenomenon. Life expectancy has shot up in recent decades, even if it appears to be stagnating in some poorer areas of the country. For men it is now a shade over seventy-nine, with the female equivalent at nearly eighty-three.[7] However, what is known as healthy life expectancy, the period during which you can live without some sort of age-related impairment, is notably smaller and has either been rising less quickly than overall life expectancy (for men) or falling (for women). The gap between the two figures – which roughly translates as the period during which someone is likely to require medical assistance or a form of care – is now 16.5 years for men, and 20.9 years for women.[8] Of Britons over seventy-five, almost a third say they have heart and circulatory problems, and 30 per cent report musculoskeletal conditions like arthritis or back pain.[9] This health gap affects a huge number of people. Slightly under 20 per cent of the UK population, or about 12 million people, are now aged sixty-five or over, with more than 1.5 million of these eighty-five or above.[10]

This combined shift in both mortality and morbidity is

happening around the world, with medical advances meaning many fewer people are dying from infectious diseases. There are, of course, other significant factors at play, for example changes in food production and consumption which now mean, for the first time in human history, that more people are dying from excess than malnutrition.

Someone who has seen these trends at first hand is Jonathan Valabhji, a consultant in diabetes at another leading London teaching hospital, St Mary's, who is also the NHS's spokesman on the condition. 'What we have seen is a massive change over the last few decades in terms of the type of illnesses that we're dealing with, and the demographic,' he says. Twenty years ago, Valabhji notes, his clinic for people with complications from diabetes saw relatively few old patients, for the simple reason that few survived for extended periods. 'In that era, people were having their index cardiac event – their heart attack – and dying, or at least not surviving very long after,' he says. 'Now we're not seeing that. They now happen later, and people are surviving longer, even into their eighties or nineties. That's changing the burden of disease. I'm using my clinic as an example, but it's playing out right across the sector. The net effect of all of those things is that we're seeing people live longer lives, which is a huge achievement, but they're developing conditions like diabetes with another twenty years to live, or much more than that. So we have a somewhat older population with multiple, long-term conditions.'[11]

Type 2 diabetes is often used as an example of the difficulties caused by modern, lifestyle-connected diseases, and for good reason. In the UK, one in six hospital patients have it,[12] as against one in sixteen of the general population.[13] What are likely to be conservative estimates of the medical costs put it at £2.1 billion a year in the UK, with an additional £7.7 billion in societal costs due to conditions such as amputations and blindness.[14]

Type 2 diabetes is particularly notable as a condition still generally associated with middle-aged and older people, but where the age profile has reduced. In England and Wales, there are now nearly 7,000 people under twenty-five living with it.[15] Back at King's, Martin Whyte is discussing his experiences in another element of his job, running a diabetes clinic as part of an academic role in Surrey, just outside London. 'I see this in the clinic all the time,' says Whyte. 'It used to always be the case that if you had someone in their twenties with diabetes they'd have type 1. Now you can't take that as a given. We do see lots of type 2 diabetes now, and you even hear about it in paediatric clinics. And there's loads of people in their twenties and thirties.'

Whyte says he sees many middle-aged people being admitted at King's who had believed they were healthy, but turn out to have been incubating a series of conditions, including diabetes. 'We often see the first presentation of what has clearly been there chronically, but is only just being unmasked,' he says. One of the very modern-day complications of such cases, he adds, is that some of the people who did not know they had type 2 diabetes arrive after spending months consuming large amounts of high-sugar energy drinks to try to cope with the tiredness it brings, which has just made the condition even worse.

We cannot stand still

It can be difficult to put into figures the total additional costs imposed on health services due to inactivity, not least as it is so often just one of a series of risk factors harboured by people. A study by Public Health England concluded it costs the NHS £455 million per year, while stressing this only covered direct costs and was thus a significant underestimate.[16]

Seemingly more realistic was a paper by the US government's Centers for Disease Control, which sought to work out the healthcare costs of inactivity while also accounting for the parallel risks of obesity. Merging data from more than 50,000 patient interviews and cost surveys, it found healthcare spending for inactive and insufficiently active people was on average 12.5 per cent higher, and was still 11.1 per cent more when body weight was taken into account. Overall, it said, inactivity totalled just over £100 billion extra per year in additional costs.[17] A 2016 study in *The Lancet* came up instead with what it called a 'conservatively estimated' total cost of £42 billion to medical services worldwide from activity, as well as an extra £11 billion in lost productivity.[18]

Such figures are almost too significant to properly appreciate. As another metric, Whyte estimates that around a third of all the emergency cases he sees have ailments connected to inactivity, a proportion that rises to around half if you combine this with the interlinked issue of patients who are also overweight or obese. 'It is a major, major problem,' he says. 'Absolutely – there's no doubt about it. And the increased pressure is noticeable every year.'

Added to this, Whyte says, is the fact that even if sedentary living might not be the direct cause of someone's ailment, it is likely to have worsened it: 'If you're looking at metabolic and cardiovascular conditions – and there's a huge overlap between diabetes and cardiovascular disease – inactivity is clearly a factor. Equally, with lung disease, normally when you're active you're taking deep breaths in and out, you're clearing, you're ventilating. It's almost like opening the windows and getting the dust out of a room – it cleans everything through. So if you're not active, if you're not getting that ventilation, things will settle in the lungs. You can get what's called atelectasis, which is where the lung just becomes a bit floppy, and sits down on itself. And the body doesn't like stasis. The body likes to be constantly moving, so if you have atelectasis you're much more likely to get infections.'

Kelly gives an even higher estimate for the proportion of his patients brought to the hospital with conditions caused in part from inactivity. During an interview which begins as he strides back to his office in the top levels of the hospital, me half-jogging alongside, audio recorder held hopefully in the air, Kelly spends at least five minutes verbally mulling this over. 'Now there's a question,' he begins, launching into a response that takes in subjects including eighteenth-century economist Adam Smith's ideas on the specialisation of behaviour and the legacy of Margaret Thatcher. Eventually he comes up with a figure: anything up to 60 per cent. Pausing some more, he adds: 'In fact, if I was to go through the current ward I think it would be more difficult to find patients for whom inactivity is *not* an issue. Of course, I've got a skewed population. I'm an adult physician in a central London teaching hospital with a lot of racial, economic, political and religious variation. But I can't think of one at the moment.'

Kelly is adamant that unless things change, then the NHS as he knows it, universal and free at the point of use, will not survive. 'We cannot stand still as things are,' he explains. 'And it's not even about standing still. So what gives? The short answer is: the way things are at the moment, which is fragile anyway, cannot be maintained. Our skill at keeping us alive to present later with more conditions and more medications is unsustainable. I don't say that as a failure of what we do to keep people alive. The tap is being turned on more and more and more, and no one is doing anything about the plug hole. But it's not medicine that's causing the problem, it's public health.'

Those tasked with surveying the health system from a broader perspective have reached the same conclusions. Dr Justin Varney, formerly head of adult wellbeing for Public Health England, who is now in charge of public health for the city of Birmingham, tells me: 'I think people are realising that the whole concept of an NHS and welfare state, in whatever form we have it, is completely unsustainable if a third or more of the population remain physically inactive.'

This is, he says, as much an issue of overall national economic viability as just about health services. 'The problem of inactive lives is growing, and I think we're understanding now much more clearly the direct correlation between inactivity, population health and economic sustainability,' he says. 'It's not just that being inactive contributes to over twenty-four long-term conditions, it's also that if you're inactive you're more likely to be socially isolated, you're not likely to be part of the job market and achieving your full economic potential, and although you may well be living longer in terms of total years of life, you're going to be living more of those years with ill-health and impairment, and therefore require much larger demands for social care and support, as well as not having the happiest retirement.'

The population-wide consequences of this are almost incalculable, Varney says: 'In the context that a third of kids today will see their 100th birthday, we fundamentally cannot afford to continue with the legacy of inactivity, because those children would live a life in which potentially forty years is lived with chronic disease, and that will break the system. Certainly in the context of the UK welfare state it's completely unaffordable. But also from the context of business, those people will need to remain economically in the job market well into their seventies, and in order to work you need to be physically active.'[19]

Such problems do not just affect the UK, or even similarly sedentary developed nations like the US and Australia. Fiona Bull is an inactivity expert with the World Health Organization, and was one of the co-authors of the landmark 2012 *Lancet* study which revealed how widespread it now is around the world. Bull notes that the United Nations runs regular high-level summits on the problem of lifestyle-connected diseases, particularly for poorer countries, where people are also living longer but with more ailments, many connected to the loss of activity from people's lives, whether from changed jobs or the growth of motor transport.

'The burden for non-communicable diseases is a burden that is unsustainable and will cause great pressure on the current health systems, not to mention fragile health systems in developing countries,' she says. 'You simply cannot provide enough medication and healthcare services for these chronic diseases at the volume that we are creating through the lifestyles people lead, and the failure to deal with the risk factors.'

Again, this is not just about inactivity. A range of other risks exist in various regions, for example efforts by tobacco giants to market their products in Africa amid declining sales on other continents. Children are also growing up more overweight than their parents, as well as less active, Bull notes: 'There is a clustering of risk factors in these younger age groups which is unprecedented. It's going to lead to even more diseases, which healthcare systems will be required to handle. And we can't afford it. No country can afford it.'[20]

Of Bull's four major risks for NCDs, tobacco and alcohol abuse are relatively easy to untangle. With inactivity and obesity, they are often combined, not least because of their joint contribution to one of the major chronic health burdens of the era: type 2 diabetes. As Jonathan Valabhji, who has spent nearly thirty years helping people with the condition, says: 'If you're asking me, "I've got someone with a new diagnosis of type 2 diabetes, what percentage of the determination of their onset is attributable to diet and what to exercise?" No, I can't give you that, and I don't think anyone can.'

The graph of doom

There is a second, hugely important strand to this story of inactivity and the social and economic costs it imposes on countries. This is looking after vulnerable older people, otherwise known as social care, which is simultaneously one of the most pressing and more neglected political issues of our times.

In health terms, it is simply a time-based extension of the effect of millions more people simultaneously living longer lives but developing chronic illnesses and conditions, many related to inactivity, at younger ages. At some point, many are no longer able to care for themselves.

This phenomenon is being witnessed across the world, but it is particularly acute in wealthier countries with ageing populations, such as the UK with its increasingly wide gap between healthy life expectancy and overall life expectancy. Of course, this is an average figure, and by no means every person aged over sixty-five, or even those aged over eighty-five, are unable to live independently. But millions of older people in the UK do need assistance – everything from occasional help in their own home, to regular visits, or then life in a residential care setting. In many cases the work is done by relatives, which while unpaid has a huge economic effect, as carers are often left unable to do other jobs. Some wealthier older people pay for support.

But that leaves an enormous and increasing burden on the state social care sector, provided as a legal obligation by increasingly cash-strapped councils, which have seen their central government budgets slashed in the past decade. Some of the obligations cover social care for vulnerable children, but the great majority of the cost is for older people, and it is hard to overstate how much of a financial challenge this has already become. I can remember speaking to the leader of one English council, who told me that in just five years, the costs of social care in his borough had risen by 25 per cent. Another English council, in 2018, had to formally declare it could not meet its obligations.[21] The impact of the Covid-19 pandemic on people living in care homes illustrated the strains felt on the sector, with the virus often spread between homes by agency staff working long hours in multiple locations. Councils and care providers are still awaiting a long-promised UK government plan for the sector. The situation is the same in many other countries.

The scale of this challenge was laid out a decade ago by something known – in all seriousness – as the *Barnet Graph of Doom*. Renowned by those who have heard of it as one of the more frightening PowerPoint slides ever created, it was the work of Andrew Travers, who at the time was the head of finance for Barnet council, on the northern fringes of London. The horizontal axis has a rising series of bars showing the combined cost of adult and child social care for Barnet over time, both historic and projected a decade or so into the future. The vertical axis, represented as a line, shows the total budget for the council. At some point in the 2020s, they meet. This would mean the entire budget used up for social care, with nothing left for anything else – libraries, parks, bin collections, anything.

There is, of course, a good argument that the graph represents an oversimple extrapolation of current trends, but the point is eloquent. Travers now works at another London council, Lambeth, where I talk to him. The *Graph of Doom*, he concedes with some pride, remains well known 'in rarefied circles', and caused a brief fright among ministers. 'Central government heard about it because people rang them to ask, "Is this right, is the end of the world coming?"' Travers recalls. 'Once it did get that wider currency we were keen to say that it wasn't necessarily predicting precisely what will happen. But we were trying to explain a narrative that we believe to be true, i.e. the fundamental difficulty of reducing resources and increasing demand, just to make that clear to people. And it succeeded quite well in doing that.'

Travers also makes the point that the crises in the health and social care system are not separate, in that many older people who go to hospital have to be discharged into some form of care – and if that does not exist, they cannot leave. This could soon bring a year-round shortage of hospital beds, he predicts: 'It wouldn't just be a winter NHS crisis – you might see it in the spring, and the autumn.'[22]

What is the connection to inactivity? It is because, as we'll see more fully in a later chapter, staying active as you age is a huge predictor of how likely you are to remain healthy and independent. Regular physical exertion has been shown to affect everything from strength and balance (and thus the likelihood of falling) to bone mass and cognitive ability, as well as the risks of developing all sorts of debilitating illnesses. To borrow the Ralph Paffenbarger maxim: 'Anything that gets worse as you grow older gets better when you exercise.' Or, as one public health expert once put it to me, more bluntly: 'I tell people, "Being active throughout your life is about being able to get to the loo on time in your old age." They can get their heads around that.'

Numerous studies have backed this up. One ongoing US-based

project reported in 2014 on older people and their ability to walk unaided, a key factor of independent living. It involved around 1,600 people aged seventy-plus whose fitness was tested as low, but could still walk 400 metres. They were split into two groups, one of which was put through low-level physical activity, with the other given workshops on better ageing and some stretching exercises. In a follow-up just two and a half years later, significantly more of the latter group had problems walking longer distances than those who had undergone the activity programme.[23]

The results reinforce one of the lessons I have picked up while researching this book: if you are ever a test subject in a public health trial, and one of the intervention options involves physical activity, do whatever you can to end up in that group. These decisions are usually randomised, but try to bribe a researcher to fix it. You'll benefit in the end.

Better without medicine

As we've seen already in the book, simply telling people they should move more is not enough. The same is true even when the people telling them are doctors. For all that doctors are often the first person to break to someone the consequences they face due to decades of inactive living, even the most passionate physician cannot single-handedly dismantle the societal pressures people face, assuming they had the time.

Asked if it can be a depressing experience to simply help people manage preventable conditions, Martin Whyte agrees. 'I do find that,' he says. 'I put it as a sort of pyramid, standing on its tip. You've got this patient at the bottom, at the tip, with this extraordinary array of forces bearing down on them that could make them have conditions like diabetes. From the top you've got transportation policy, the plethora of shops selling fast food; you've got advertising. To expect me to make significant inroads on that individual at the bottom of that enormous pyramid – to blithely say something like, "You need to follow the Mediterranean diet, or move more" – that's futile. There's much bigger forces at work. So I do find it very frustrating. It's almost to the point of nihilism: you can't expect much traction from that one-to-one clinical encounter.'

His colleague, Phil Kelly, presents a similar picture when asked if it can feel exhausting to encounter the same preventable conditions again and again: 'That's an interesting one. Because you're right: because we have demonstrated, even within Europe, that we don't have to have things the way they are. You can have a public health approach. It doesn't have to be a totalitarian shove into the gymnasium.' He pauses for a while: 'But now I'm thinking – maybe I'm not worried enough. My job is to make sense of a certain group of things, and perhaps to keep doing it I have to see the glass as half full, or it would be very difficult to get through the hours until you're next exposed to the difficulties of human existence. So undoubtedly I get frustrated, that's a no-brainer.'

The issues, Kelly notes, also reach into areas such as the wide inequalities of income and opportunity in the highly mixed southeast London district where he works. 'I think we could have not monetised school playing fields over generations,' he says. 'We could have completely invested in other ways to transport ourselves around our cities. We could have normalised exercise in youth and teenage years, to make it extremely easy and normal to be engaged in some form of social exercise. It could be social contact as well. I think we have had the opportunity to do that. So do I get frustrated that we might have made different choices? Yes.

'And if I think about the disparity in opportunity between

people, I've no problem if by circumstance or luck or nous you have more of what society deems important, and you can send your children to places with magnificent sporting facilities. But is the net appropriately spread for the others? I don't think it is. That frustrates me – why does the child in Peckham not have the same exposure to activity as every other child?'

Such thoughts are not lost on politicians and senior policy-makers, even if they are less likely to delve into such politically contentious areas. There is, nonetheless, an argument that health services could be doing more to raise awareness of the problems caused by inactivity. The NHS's latest long-term strategic plan,[24] unveiled at the start of 2019, contains fervent calls for more pre-ventative public health action, but little in the way of specifics. In contrast, the whizz-bang world of high-tech, curative medicine is spelled out in much more detail, with promises of genomic screen-ing, digital consultations with doctors and other innovations.

In part, this is perhaps connected to the expectations of a public still more used to doctors handing out medicines to treat their ailments than offering advice on how to prevent them in the first place. Jonathan Valabhji says he believes this is gradually changing: 'I've spent most of the last twenty-nine years sitting opposite patients in one setting or another, and one really tangible shift is that many people are now open to or even prefer the suggestion of a lifestyle intervention to do something, versus a tablet. Some people still have the attitude of problems being solved ideally on a prescription pad – that's the model of the health service that many of our population hold dear. But if we tackle the younger and younger ages of onset of long-term conditions, and the costs to the NHS, we need to put a stronger spotlight on prevention. That's very much the narrative.'

During my day at King's I spot something in common about the offices of Kelly and Whyte – both doctors have folded bicycles tucked away in a corner, their regular transport into work. 'It might take me slightly longer, but it's predictable,' Whyte says. 'There's no stress about missing the train, or the train being late.' He admits to being 'quite militant' about wanting people to be more active, advocating warning signs on lifts: 'They would be like the ones on cigarette packets: "This lift will damage your health." We're on the fourth floor, and I see people getting in the lift and they go up one floor, sometimes even down.' Whyte bursts into appalled laughter: 'It's terrible!'

It is one thing for middle-class, well-educated doctors to know about the risks of sedentary living, but quite another for them to have the time to offer advice, and yet another thing in turn for patients to heed the guidance, and then continue to do so long-term in a world seemingly designed around inactivity.

Some are looking for new ways to spread the message. Andrew Boyd, the lead on physical activity for the body that represents UK family doctors, the Royal College of General Practitioners, is pushing for a series of innovations. One would be for GPs to routinely work from standing desks, giving them a chance to explain the benefits to presumably surprised patients. Another would remove the ubiquitous electronic sign systems in surgery waiting rooms. Instead, doctors would walk from their office and call people in – giving the GP invaluable exertion, as well as a chance to discuss why they are doing it. 'GPs can't do everything – and in particular they can't make it easier for people to walk or cycle places, or not have a desk job,' Boyd tells me. 'But too often people don't even realise how dangerous their lifestyles are.'

One recent change, Boyd says, is for time-pressed family doctors to be helped on these issues by specialist non-medical staff called 'social prescribers', who can spend longer with patients and help them find lifestyle interventions, whether based around activity or anything else, which could improve their health without the need for more medication. 'There's estimates that about a quarter of the people we see have non-medical issues, or at least an issue that could be managed with non-medical interventions,' Boyd notes.

Some pioneering doctors' practices have tried solutions like prescribing people membership of a local bicycle share scheme, or suggesting they try their local Parkrun, the fast-growing, non-competitive social running movement we'll hear more about later in the book. Boyd says the social prescribers' most common solution is for people to simply walk more: 'It's free, and you can combine it into your day. It's whatever works for that individual, and that's why it has to take the form of a con-versation – what would help someone do the sorts of things they want to do? That's why you can't fit it into a ten-minute GP's conversation when you've already dealt with their acute issue and any medication issue.'[25]

A similar lack of time and resources affects hospital doctors in helping patients with lifestyle advice. The NHS has a group support programme to help people with diabetes, particularly type 2, which covers physical activity, as well as diet and other areas. But according to Martin Whyte, a combination of mixed availability and limited motivation means only around 5 per cent of his patients take part.

Others are prompted to take action themselves, Whyte notes: 'You often get people who come in with a heart attack and type 2 diabetes. They have the heart problem and the diabetes diagnosed at the same time. They might have been inactive or overweight, but they felt healthy and thought they were – it can be a big shock for people. Some get depressed but for some they want to turn their life around. I've had people at my diabetes clinic where the transformation is amazing. But if it's based around something like a gym or running, you have to ask – will it last in the long term? There are huge pressures and forces at play, and I don't think the NHS is the place that can fight against them. We see the net results, which is the presentations through the front door, or in the clinics. And it's huge.'

It seems that the response has to begin with politicians, not doctors. As Phil Kelly sits in his office, he again ponders one of my questions, this time whether the looming crisis in the NHS will eventually force government ministers to start making bold choices. Eventually he replies: 'No, is the short answer. You may say, we will get so close to the point of cataclysm and then we will draw back. But what of many points so far was not cataclysmic? What are we waiting for? The short-term reward from not providing playing fields for schools, or not having a reasonable public health approach to diet in children – there's too much to gain from ignoring it. We're all guilty of short-termism. And the official response so far is a bit weak.' Kelly sits back in his chair, sighs, and then grins: 'Of course, you could have just caught me after a bad ward round.'

For a slightly more hopeful note on which to end the chapter, let us return down the corridor to Whyte's office, where he is describing what he says is perhaps the biggest individual success story he has seen in his diabetes clinic. It was, Whyte recalls, a middle-aged man with type 2 diabetes.

'By this point he had been coming to the clinic off and on for several years. He was on all sorts of medication, and he was overweight,' Whyte explains. 'With this clinic, when patients come in, they get blood taken and we get immediate results, which I see before the patients – it helps us understand how they've been managing their diabetes for the previous few months. Anyway, this time there was a sudden, massive improvement in this man's readings. He told me he now wasn't taking any medication either.

'I said, "That's incredible – what happened?" He said he'd got a job as a postman. It was just through walking on the delivery round, especially up and down hills, that everyday activity dramatically transformed his diabetes. It stuck in my head – it was such an amazing thing. I thought: if only everyone in the clinic could get a job as a postman. It was profound. Medicine works, but it's much better to do it without medicine.'

As we will see in the next chapter, for most people it is, sadly, not that simple. Without something like a job which guarantees daily movement, you are significantly more reliant on the built environment around you, one which often seems to conspire to make physical exertion as difficult as possible.

If there is a message for this chapter, perhaps for the entire book, it is that for all the wonders achieved by modern medicine, without concerted, significant, interventionist action at a national political level, the sorts of universal health and social care systems many millions of people take for granted could effectively be gone within a generation. The hugely optimistic example of Martin Whyte's revitalised, drugs-free postman simply demonstrates the overriding need to help make lifestyles built around activity a more normal thing. Multiply his example by the millions, and so much of the problem goes away.

Next steps:

Type 2 diabetes is the chronic medical condition perhaps most closely linked with inactive living, and many people do not know they could be at risk. Diabetes UK has an excellent, and very simple, web questionnaire, which uses factors like your waist size, height, weight, family history of diabetes and ethnicity to instantly assess your likely chances of developing it. Search for "Diabetes UK risk score" to find out yours.

5

Towns and Cities on a Human Scale

It is over an hour into a chat I had promised Jan Gehl would take considerably less time, but the Danish architect, now eighty-three, is still animatedly explaining the ideas he pioneered about the way towns and cities should be designed for the needs of their inhabitants, and particularly the ways in which these people can move around under their own power.

Leaning forward in his chair in the light-filled meeting room of his eponymous architectural practice in Copenhagen, where he is still a regular presence despite officially being retired, Gehl puts one hand vertically on the table, the downward-facing fingers closed into a stationary block, to indicate a slab of a building. 'This is easy to communicate in still photos, and easy to study,' he tells me in his precise, lightly accented English. Gehl then starts wiggling the hand's fingers to show people walking around: 'This is much more complicated to study. And this is complicated to communicate. But it is very important. And that is what I've been involved in – making the people who use cities visible for politicians, and for my fellow colleagues around the world.'

Gehl cheerfully describes himself as 'an anti-modernist and anti-motorist', someone who has spent more than half a century rejecting the idea that the urban domain should be seen through the prism of monolithic tower blocks and offices, and the highways snaking around them. Instead, he believes, towns and cities need to be focused on the everyday movements and interactions of human beings, travelling at human-powered speeds. Gehl's philosophy is summed up by the hugely evocative, almost poetic title of the 1971 book in which he presented his ideas: *Life Between Buildings*.[1]

When he first qualified as an architect, Gehl tells me, it was 1960, perhaps the heyday of modernism, when towns and cities were being reshaped according to a template in which near-universal car use was assumed as the default. At the time he was a true believer. So what changed? It was, Gehl tells me, meeting his wife, who is a psychologist.

'I was meant to start with all these high-rise suburbs and freeways,' Gehl recounts. 'But she and her friends, they kept saying, "Why are you architects not interested in people? Have you thought about why your professors go out at four o'clock in the morning to take photos of their various monuments? It's to be certain there will be no people in the foreground to distract the students during the lectures. Because we know, of course, that if there are people in the foreground, they will start to look at them. Because the biggest interest of people is other people."'

Gehl and his wife went to Italy for six months to examine the street layouts and piazzas of the Renaissance-built towns and cities and see how they helped the natural flow of pedestrians. He then returned to Denmark to study the psychology of housing. 'I had this joke that when I was at university we heard nothing about people, and so I had to go back to forget everything they told me,' he says. 'We had to sit down at square one and start to see how people used architecture, how people used cities, and gradually accumulate knowledge about what were the important factors. Many of my colleagues thought I was crazy. They said, "You're ruining your career!"'

Gehl's colleagues need not have worried. He is now regularly lauded as one of the most influential urban thinkers of the modern era, with expertise that has been sought by cities as disparate as Sydney, Moscow and New York. His programme to make Sydney greener and less car-dominated, with pedestrianised streets, bike lanes and a new light rail system, saw him become only the second Dane to receive the key to the city, its highest honour, after Jørn Utzon, another architect, who designed its famous opera house.

Perhaps the city which best epitomises Gehl's philosophy is his own, where decades of human-friendly planning mean more than 40 per cent of all commuting trips in Copenhagen are now made by bike. Gehl opens his laptop to show me a photograph: in 2017, to mark the city's 850th anniversary, Copenhagen's council put up posters of the ten residents judged to have most shaped it over that period, with Gehl among them. 'They had the founder, and king this and king that, and Hans Christian Andersen,' Gehl recalls with obvious delight. 'And then me – they said I was responsible for Copenhagen today. I rushed all over the city to see the poster on bus stops.'

Gehl has a mischievously dry sense of humour, telling me that because of his age he has to turn down most invitations to appear at overseas events: 'I say now that if they want me for sure they just have to hand me a medal. That's my principle. If they want to do something in that direction, I come.'

But his pride in his work is obvious: 'I can say, after fifty years, that now we know how to make nice cities for people. I have had the chance to formulate the principles, to study the subject, to find out how things work, what you can do, and be able to do it in a number of places. I am able to see life here in my own city, like in Melbourne, Sydney, in Moscow, with these ideas being realised and used, and see that they have a tremendous impact on the quality of life. It is a privilege to be as old as I am.'[2]

Before looking at what all this means in practice, let's take a step back to consider why it matters so much. The ideas for which Gehl has battled are central to perhaps the most important element of the modern world's unspoken war against everyday activity. It is one thing for governments and anxious health officials to urge people to move more in their lives. But when so much of the built environment makes this task, at best, much less convenient than it should be and, at worst, virtually impossible, it's no wonder so little changes.

This chapter is about activity in the public realm, whether on roads, in squares, streets and other spaces, as well as inside communal buildings and, perhaps most importantly, the way we travel to, from and between all of these. It is a story, in many ways, about infrastructure, which might appear at first a somewhat technocratic, even dull, subject, but holds an enormous influence over vast areas of most people's lives.

One thing is clear: if someone is to meet the universally recommended 150 minutes of moderate exertion a week as part of their routine life, rather than formal exercise, then both practicality and the mechanics of energy expenditure dictate that a good proportion of it will come from time spent outside the home. And for many people, a significant proportion of this will involve active travel, whether walking or cycling.

Currently, this overriding need for human-speed movement happens in an environment shaped by humanity, largely around the needs of motor vehicles. The world has now passed the point in which a majority of people live in towns and cities, with the estimated global urbanisation rate now around 55 per cent.[3] In the UK, even though considerably less than 90 per cent of land is built on,[4] 83 per cent of the population is urban.[5]

Unlike other areas of modern life which have helped push out everyday movement, the urban status quo is deeply problematic for a number of reasons. While no one is really suggesting that people do away with labour-saving appliances in the home, when it comes to the takeover of virtually all human-powered travel by the motor vehicle, it is a different story. This is not to say cars should not exist, simply that they are not necessarily needed for the countless millions of tiny journeys they undertake every day. Such mass car use causes enormous damage in a series of areas entirely separate from activity, everything from choking air pollution to dangerous, socially disconnected cities, plus of course a significant role in the global, existential threat of the climate emergency.

Directly relevant to this book, however, is the fact that the hegemony of cars hugely restricts the ability of people to walk and cycle, which are where the real gains can be made in terms of both energy consumed and exertion levels reached. To look back to the study we saw in the first chapter about the activity levels of various home tasks done manually or by machine, it found that washing dishes by hand, something that many people still do now, burns up around 110 calories per hour. In contrast, a hypothetical brief walk to a job uses about double that, while stair climbing goes beyond 250 calories an hour. The study didn't include cycling, but if I take the estimated calorie count from my borrowed wrist-worn fitness tracker, the near-twenty-minute ride from my home to my temporary writing base – some of which is, admittedly, up a relatively steep hill – involves an outflow of just under 180 calories. We are suddenly over 500 calories an hour. That is a lot of energy expended.

Active travel has another advantage. It is the very definition of incidental activity, that concept so beloved of public health advocates, where movement becomes a part of life which is happening anyway. When I cycle for transport, the calories burned and other associated health boosts are hugely welcome. But they're not the main reason I do it. I cycle around a city because it is reliable, rapid and has the happy ability to deliver me to my destination within a minute or so of when I expected, often with a smile on my face.

The 40 per cent gain

It's worth immediately stressing that whether or not they are a secondary concern, the health dividends of active travel can be enormous. In earlier chapters we saw the many benefits of walking, particularly at a brisk pace. This remains true when people do it for everyday transport. One UK study from 2017, using data from the huge and ongoing government-backed Biobank public health project, tracked more than 250,000 people across the country over five years. When other variables were factored out, it found that people who walked to work had almost a 30 per cent lower chance of suffering from heart disease in that time.

That said, the benefits really start to multiply if you get on a bicycle. The same Biobank study concluded that those who commuted by bike had even lower odds of heart disease, with the risks cut by 50 per cent. The cyclists also saw the same reduction in risk for cancer, and had an overall 40 per cent lower chance of dying during the study period. In contrast, for people who commuted by foot, there was no measurable benefit with cancer or overall mortality rates.[6]

The 40 per cent reduced mortality statistic is particularly resonant, as it exactly matches the findings of the Danish study into cycle commuting I quoted at the very start of this book as an example of the wonder-drug qualities of regular activity. That Danish research was published in 2000,[7] and for years was routinely wheeled out as the go-to academic paper for vividly illustrating the marvels of activity. And now its findings have been replicated, precisely, in another country.

You could spend a long time reading similar scientific paeans to the benefits of cycling. The reason why it appears to be so health-bringing is the fact that riding a bike almost invariably pushes you into the realm of moderate, or even vigorous, exertion. The threshold for moderate is a mere three METs, and while the calculations for what constitutes such an effort on a bike varies between riders, it's generally seen as pretty leisurely, even below 10mph. To reach the six METs needed for vigorous activity is not a huge amount faster, with some tables suggesting even as little as 12mph could do it. And if you suddenly find yourself sprinting for a green traffic light, or riding up a steep hill, the MET total is suddenly into ten or more.

Even if your bike-riding approach is notably sedate, you have to try fairly hard to not reach at least a moderate level, particularly when climbing any sort of incline. As one public health academic half-joked to me, the difference between walking and cycling is that with the former, anyone can have a lazy day and stroll at about two METs, whereas if you went that slowly on a bike you would probably fall off.

To try to find out how strenuous a fairly regular cycle commute can be, I decided to enlist the help of a test subject: me. In non-coronavirus times, I make the three-and-a-half-mile trip between my south London home and Westminster maybe four or five times a week. No one would mistake this for sport or exercise. I use a heavy, practical bike, with hub gears and a huge basket at the front into which I can throw my bag. I ride in office clothes, which not only saves the effort of bringing in a change of outfit, but spares me having to experience the single, generally pretty grimy, men's shower in the media enclave of the Houses of Parliament.

Because my borrowed fitness watch only arrived after lock-down, the commute had to be replicated using what was then my government-sanctioned daily exercise. I tried to make it as accurate as possible, riding at a pace that didn't make me overly sweaty, even putting my work bag in the basket. The watch has built-in GPS and so measured the distance and speed, as well as tracking my heart rate over both journeys. The results were illuminating, not least in highlighting the point about how useful a cycle commute is for getting you somewhere roughly when you expect it. The outward trip ended up taking me seventeen minutes and twenty-two seconds. The return was quicker – by precisely three seconds. That's predictability.

In terms of health benefits, the heart rate data indicated I spent pretty much all the journey exerting myself moderately or vigorously. The watch, made by the US firm Garmin, splits the efforts you make into five 'zones' based on your maximum heart rate. According to the company's charts, even zone one indicates an exertion of between 50 per cent and 60 per cent of the maximum, which still officially counts as moderate. To be overly cautious I excluded my zone-one time, and took moderate activity to be zone two (60 per cent to 70 per cent of maximum), with vigorous as three or above. Even calculated like this the amounts stacked up gratifyingly. The there-and-back total was about five and a half minutes of moderate activity, and a bit over twenty-five minutes of vigorous exertion.

If you remember from earlier chapters, while the recommended minimum amount of moderate activity needed to maintain health is half an hour, five times a week, for vigorous effort this halves, to just fifteen minutes a day. My sample commute alone seemingly gives me almost two days' worth. That's not bad as an added extra for something I mainly do because it is reliable and fun.

This is, of course, a study with a sample size of precisely one, with the subject also being the researcher. There's an argument that as someone who has cycled for years, I'm perhaps more likely than average to exert myself, even when trying to avoid an excessive sweat. I also have to confess that on the final section of the return leg that day, riding up the gradual hill to the street where I live, I tried to keep up with a much younger rider on a lightweight bike. But, again, that's one of the benefits of cycle commuting – you do sometimes end up trying harder than you planned.

There is one, final question. How fit does this very routine regime leave me? One answer, provided by the activity watch, is my resting heart rate, for which it helpfully gives a seven-day average. At time of writing it tells me mine is forty-eight beats a minute. This is a fairly broad gauge, but the general metric is that resting rates below sixty are rare unless you are pretty active. So that's a good first sign.

Before I sound too complacent, I must introduce another measure. Just before the lockdown I put myself through a much more rigorous regime at the sports science department of Roehampton University, the base for Dr Richard Mackenzie, whom we met in Chapter 2. This is a VO2 max test, which measures maximum oxygen uptake. With a score expressed in millilitres of oxygen absorbed per kilo of body weight per minute, it is seen as a good gauge of aerobic fitness, even if its precise worth is endlessly debated in academic circles.

It is not a comfortable process. It is done by what is termed a 'ramp test' – basically, putting your body under ever greater strain until you have to give up, slumped and wheezing. I did mine on a stationary bike, where I had to produce higher and higher watts of pedalling power over time, all the while with a clammy mask covering my face, connected to a machine. It was not made any easier by the fact I did it while suffering from a slight chest infection. And yes, I am perhaps getting my excuses in early.

When the results came back my score was forty, which for my age puts me in a category – depending on which chart you check – just between 'good' and 'excellent'. And yet I was pretty disappointed. Why? It's because I had done the same test a few years earlier and scored fifty-three, which put me in the wonderfully named class of 'superior'. At the time, my bike commute was roughly twice as long – I was still based at my newspaper's headquarters rather than parliament – and I did other activities, like swimming.

This was, in a weird way, perhaps a wake-up call. Yes, all the evidence shows that even my fairly brief and routine commute brings me almost incalculable health benefits, and keeps me notably fitter than the great majority of middle-aged men. But, as we saw in earlier chapters, one of the many amazing things about physical exertion is that the health dividends almost never stop – more is just about always even better. That is perhaps one minor consideration before you integrate an activity like cycling into your everyday life – it can all become a bit addictive.

This is the point at which a sceptic might say: what good is an 'excellent' or even 'superior' VO2 max score if you end up dead? The biggest single reason cited for why so few people cycle in the UK is safety, particularly perceived safety. Such concerns are hugely understandable, and play an enormous part in low levels of active travel. At the same time, however, they should be put into proportion and context.

As we heard at the start of the book, an estimated 100,000 people a year in the UK die early because of health issues connected to inactive living.[8] In contrast, over the same period around 100 cyclists are killed on the country's roads.[9] Yes, this is in part because of the relatively small numbers who cycle, and the figure could and should be less. Exact comparisons are difficult, but the best estimates suggest that cycling in the Netherlands, with its thousands of miles of separated bike lanes and two wheeled–friendly road culture, is between three and four times safer than in the UK.[10]

Even so, however, the odds are still very much with you. UK government figures show a serious injury or fatality happens, on average, every million miles cycled. A 2010 study by Dutch academics attempted to balance the health benefits of activity from cycling against the various risks, not just crashes but also the effects of air pollution. In the Netherlands, with its many miles of safe cycle lanes, as you might expect the balance was very firmly pro-bike, with the benefits-to-risks ratio calculated at nine to one. But even when the UK's less safe roads for cyclists were factored in, this fell only to seven to one. That is still pretty overwhelming.[11]

However, it takes more than citing a few statistics to persuade people to cycle. One innovative study by Professor Rachel Aldred, a UK academic who is a leading expert on why people do and do not ride bikes for transport, involved trying to separate out the data on deaths and injuries from the lived experience of those actually getting around on two wheels. Her eloquently titled *Near Miss Project* asked participants around the UK to pick a day when they were going to cycle and then fill out an online diary about what happened. More than 80 per cent of those who took part recorded at least one frightening experience, ranging from a too-close overtake to much more serious incidents.

On average, people faced an event deemed 'very scary' once every week, with the vast majority connected to the actions of drivers.[12]

This is the context within which the near-unbelievable health dividends of regular cycling must be placed. Many people buy a bike with the best intentions of using it daily, but give up when a driver decides to carelessly skim them at 40mph. The same is even true for walking, even if the primary barriers are different. Pedestrian deaths and injuries are a reality, with more than forty pedestrians a year in Britain killed by vehicles on pavements.[13] The UK is among just a handful of European nations where pedestrian injuries have risen in recent years.[14] As I've had to stress more or less throughout this book, in virtually every area of physical activity, there are much greater factors in play than personal willpower and motivation.

To invite or to repel

So how did we end up here? Jan Gehl's self-description as being 'anti-motorist' as well as an anti-modernist is telling, because the post-war rise of the planned, inorganic city was as much about the cars as the buildings. Three years after Gehl left university as a fresh-faced and obedient advocate of the new consensus, the UK saw the publication of what was, in retrospect, one of the most malignly influential publications of the era. *Traffic in Towns*[15] first came out in 1963 as a planning report, but achieved the rare feat for such a document of becoming so popular it was later issued as a paperback book. Written by Colin Buchanan, an engineer and town planner, it expressed some concern at the rising tide of motor traffic but concluded this was the future, and thus many more roads must be built. Buchanan wondered briefly about the idea of also constructing bike routes, but dismissed this, saying it was 'a moot point' whether there would realistically be many cyclists remaining a few years down the line.

This was the era when countries around Europe, as well as the USA, were embracing car culture, with entire historic districts of cities flattened to make way for urban motorways and ringroads. This influx of motor vehicles brought a resultant drop in active travel, and a hugely increasing death toll as these new drivers interacted with the unprotected road users who still tried to brave the streets. A handful of places fought back. In the early 1970s, a prominent Dutch journalist, whose six-year-old daughter had been killed by a speeding driver as she cycled to school, launched a campaign called *Stop de Kindermoord*, or *Stop the Child Murders*,[16] sparking a campaign of civil disobedience in the Netherlands which directly led to successive governments reshaping the nation's roads. Denmark, too, saw mass protests slightly later.

In most other countries, however, Buchanan's vision of car-only personal urban transport largely came true, with significant knock-on effects for people's physical lives, not all of them obvious. One 2007 study assessed various neighbourhoods in the Australian city of Adelaide on how friendly to walking they were. It found that even after accounting for other variables, women who lived in low-walkability areas watched significantly more television than those in places where walking was easier. The same was not found for men, a difference the authors said could be connected to factors such as men being less concerned about, for example, the traffic danger of low-walkability streets.[17]

Another study in Melbourne discovered that a walkable neighbourhood was one of the strongest factors in whether or not children travelled to school on foot or by bike, rather than being driven by a parent, and that this in turn played a big part in whether they were active in other areas of their life.[18]

So what constitutes a neighbourhood in which people might be more tempted to get out of the car and walk – even to a bus stop or train station – or cycle? The answer combines the most practical of engineering measures with something much more esoteric, something almost between philosophy and activism.

For example, Jan Gehl's architectural practice is on Vesterbrogade, one of central Copenhagen's busiest streets, and when I walked to his office it was packed with motor vehicles. But on either side of the vehicle lanes are broad cycle routes, separated from the traffic with a kerb, and then another step up to the pavement. Along the middle of the road is a narrow, cobbled median strip, allowing pedestrians to cross one lane of traffic at a time.

Gehl is passionate about the ability of people on foot to be able to meander around the city as they choose, and not have to walk 200 metres to wait at a dedicated pedestrian crossing. He is particularly scathing about the idea, ubiquitous in the UK but unknown in Copenhagen, of having to press a button to activate a pedestrian green light. 'It's a human right to get across the street,' he fumes. 'It's not something you should apply for. It's only in Britain, and British-dominated areas like India and Australia, where you find this idea. If you want a lively and good city you should be able to cross almost at will, which is why in Copenhagen we have this median.'

Gehl's mantra is that the urban environment should 'invite' people to cycle or walk, make it obvious and appealing. *Life Between Buildings* spells this out in a series of choices: 'To assemble or disperse; to integrate or segregate; to invite or repel.' The book urges readers to reimagine towns and cities in their traditional purpose, a place for people to wander and roam, where encounters with others are usually unprompted and serendipitous, where children can spot friends playing outside and go to join them, in safety. It stresses the fundamental human instinct of being interested in other people. One fascinating study mentioned in the book recounts how researchers tried to examine how many people looked into the various window displays along Strøget, Copenhagen's pedestrianised main shopping street, only to discover that the most popular thing to look at was a construction site – but only when the workers were there. People were the key, not things. 'That life between buildings is a self-reinforcing process also helps to explain why many new housing developments seem so lifeless and empty,' the book explains. 'Many things go on, to be sure, but both people and events are so spread out in time and space that the individual activities almost never get a chance to grow together to larger, more meaningful and inspiring sequences of events.'[19]

Gehl has spent years finessing an opposite approach in his work reshaping cities. One vignette he recounts about the ways a more human-friendly urban landscape can improve how people both move around and interact is his work in Moscow. There, he tells me, his emphasis on useable public space proved so successful in prompting the types of accidental interactions inherent to a successful city that it was the catalyst for many new romances, and he is now officially credited with starting a Moscow baby boom.

Many of the practical details of this approach are set out in *Soft City*,[20] a recent book by David Sim, who is now the creative director of Gehl's architectural practice. Packed with example photographs of temptingly liveable urban neighbourhoods – almost none of which appear to be in the UK – Sim, who is himself Scottish, explains the vital role of spaces through which people can intuitively walk and spontaneously mix. Thus, land around apartment blocks should be a contained enclosure which feels communal, not a windy hinterland that belongs to no one.

These blocks should have multiple entrances for easy pedestrian access, and ground floors filled with cafés and shops, rather than blank-faced offices, so people have a reason to congregate. One-way streets are frowned on, not just because they encourage more rapid driving speeds, but because they lose the intuitive sense of public transport, with buses unable to run on the same road in both directions.

There is an important directive to encourage walking: the pavement should be effectively continuous, with pedestrians having automatic right of way at minor junctions, rather than turning cars. The book asks: 'Why should pedestrians on a main thoroughfare have to stop and wait at every single side street when the vehicles travelling in the same direction don't have to?' It is a fair point.

In the UK, the city that has perhaps the most ambitious plans to start moving towards a model of more active living is Greater Manchester, which aims to construct more than 1,000 miles of safe, connected walking and cycling routes in the next few years. Running the project is Chris Boardman, the former Olympic and Tour de France cyclist who went on to set up his own very successful bike company, before becoming an eloquent spokesman for better everyday cycling. In 2017 he was tempted out of what sounds like an enjoyable semi-retirement by the mayor of Manchester, Andy Burnham, with a brief to transform the city.

While the centre of Manchester has acquired a series of new pedestrianised squares and shopping streets in recent years, it is still criss-crossed by roads packed with traffic, and encircled by a busy ring road, part of which is a classic 1960s example of an elevated urban motorway, the Mancunian Way. When I meet Boardman in a bustling café on one of these new pedestrian plazas, a short walk from his office building, he explains that the hope is to create a network of cycling and walking routes that will, in a Jan Gehl style, invite people to use them. 'If you take anyone from Manchester and stand them on a street in Denmark or Holland and say, "Which do you prefer, for you and for your kids?", they'll say, "This,"' he says. 'And who wouldn't? So nobody's got a problem with the destination. That's your starting point. It's about how you move things.'

Boardman's wish is for people driving on their commute to look out of the car window, see others cycling or walking, and then decide that would be a better solution. 'It's not just about safety,' he says. 'It's got to look easy. If it's not the easiest solution, or at least as easy as what they're doing now – driving – then why would they change?' Boardman's template for any proposed scheme in the new bike and walking network is 'whether a competent twelve-year-old' could use it. He indicates the packed café: 'It's got to be understandable by anybody in this room. For a twelve-year-old, a pensioner, anyone.'[21]

To an extent, the practicalities of how you achieve such a transformation move into the formal mechanics of city design, which is slightly outside the scope of this book. But the most important thing to remember is that none of this is magic, or untested, or in doubt. A city planner in the UK only has to look a small distance across the North Sea to places like Copenhagen, or to Utrecht, which prides itself as being the most cycle-friendly city in the Netherlands, and where about 60 per cent of all trips in the centre happen by bike.[22] These places have been planning for better cycling and walking for decades, and wherever you look, the principles are pretty much the same.

One fundamental idea dictates that on busier streets with more rapid motor traffic, cyclists need a protected route, a kerb-separated lane where the safety is continuous, for example with bike-only traffic signals at junctions. That is perhaps the more straightforward element. On smaller roads, particularly residential ones, the necessity is to greatly slow down motor traffic to no more than 20mph, ideally less, through a combination of clever street design, robust enforcement and, over years, a change in the traffic culture. Some Dutch residential streets make the point abundantly clear by putting up signs saying, 'Cars are guests'.

Along with this – and it is here that some British politicians tend to have a mild fit of the vapours – must come changes to make driving less convenient for small, urban trips. A common approach is known as modal filtering, where certain streets are made access-only for cars, using separated bollards through which cyclists and pedestrians can easily pass. Thus, a journey to a local shop might take ten minutes on a bike but significantly longer in a car, nudging people into being active. The reduction in vehicle traffic also makes the streets more appealing for walking and play.

As with Jan Gehl's approach, such very practical engineering measures must be combined with a more generally different way of looking at things. The official Dutch government road design manual, something of a 388-page secular bible for those who push for active travel,[23] is based around a holistic concept called *duurzaam veilig*, or sustainable safety. One of its principles is the idea that humans are flawed, and make mistakes, and that the infrastructure surrounding them should be suitably forgiving. When you are trying to tempt out unprotected humans amid a world of speeding, two-tonne metal boxes, this is arguably as important an idea as any.

When stated this way, it all seems completely obvious, and fairly easy to implement. And yet many governments still seem incapable of doing it. To take one example, many continental European cities achieve David Sim's prescription of allowing pedestrians uninterrupted flow across side streets through the basic intervention of painting zebra crossings on every such junction. Chris Boardman wants to do this in Manchester, but at the time I spoke to him, he was battling against central government scepticism, as this has never previously been done on UK roads – although, as Boardman points out, it already does exist in the country, in virtually every supermarket car park.

A war on cars

There is generally a point during any discussion about promoting active travel when someone will pipe up to say, 'Ah, but what about my granny – is she meant to walk and cycle everywhere?' A slightly trite response might be to point out that if said granny lived in the Netherlands she might well do that anyway, given the sheer number of older Dutch people who get about by bike, with almost a fifth of those aged sixty-five and over still cycling every day.[24]

But to reiterate the earlier point, no one is arguing for an absolute ban on cars, just ways to make them less of a default choice for shorter trips, which make up the great majority in the UK. A fifth of all journeys of any sort are less than a mile long, a distance very easily managed on foot and the matter of around five minutes of cycling. And yet 20 per cent of these happen in a car. Almost 40 per cent of trips of two miles or less take place by motor vehicle.[25]

All this illustrates the scope for extra activity when it comes to everyday travel. To take another example, census data tells us that almost half the commutes in England and Wales are less than three miles each way, about 20 million trips a day.[26] Imagine if just 10 per cent of these could be made on foot or by bike – that would be 2 million people reaching their 150-minutes-a-week threshold and well beyond. The gains for health and happiness would be astonishing. In one of the papers from the previously mentioned 2012 edition of *The Lancet* on inactivity, the authors analysed data from earlier Danish research to calculate that even in this bike-friendly nation, if all current non-cyclists started to cycle, this would prevent 12,000 early deaths a year through less ill-health, as balanced against around thirty extra deaths on the roads.[27]

Another possibility for our hypothetical grandmother would be that she invested in an electric-assist bicycle, or e-bike, a relatively new innovation which has a formidable potential to change the way people travel, especially those facing slightly longer or hillier trips, or for people who don't feel up to using a traditional bike. These are hugely popular in some countries, accounting for about 40 per cent of all new bike sales in the Netherlands,[28] where they are popular with older riders. Various studies have also shown that e-bikes are particularly appealing to people who would not see themselves, traditionally, as a cyclist. They can also be beneficial for those with impairments or disabilities, sometimes in the form of e-trikes, or handcycles with electric assist.

In the UK there remains a slight, residual idea that e-bikes are almost a form of cheating. And it is an inescapable truth that if you are on an e-bike this is not entirely human-powered motion. Even with the fairly weedy 250-watt power limit on the motor, which under British law must cut out above 15mph, e-bikes do offer particular help with the more strenuous parts of cycling, like riding up hills or getting going when a traffic light turns green. That is why they can be so practical in tempting people out of cars. It is much more possible to commute in everyday clothes on an e-bike, without arriving a panting, sweaty mess. But they are not electric mopeds – you still need to pedal. Additionally, e-bikes generally allow the rider to adjust how much electric oomph is provided, which can be reduced as people become more fit.

A series of studies have shown that e-bikes do thus still deliver a significant amount of physical effort. One 2019 research paper which studied 10,000 participants across seven European cities found that those who rode traditional bikes and e-bikes amassed roughly similar tallies of MET minutes of activity per week, with the lesser exertion of those with electric assist seemingly cancelled out by the fact that they tended to ride almost twice as long on average per day. It did find that people who switched from a non-electric bike to an e-bike lost some MET minutes overall, but this was around a quarter of what was gained if people moved to an e-bike from a car or public transport. 'This data suggests that e-bike use leads to substantial increases in physical activity,' the cross-Europe research team concluded.[29]

Ashley Cooper, who is a professor of physical activity and public health at Bristol University, and has spent several decades investigating ways to get people moving in their everyday lives, says e-bikes are 'probably the best physical activity intervention I've done'. Having tried out an e-bike on holiday, Cooper was so enthused he set up a project in which a group of people with type 2 diabetes were lent e-bikes to see if they could help them become more active. The results were hugely encouraging, he explains: 'We found the majority used them a reasonable amount, and fourteen of the eighteen people actually bought the bikes at the end of the study. It seems to be something which people really take to. We measured people's heart rates and it showed that riding an e-bike in terms of heart rate response is actually more energetic than walking. It's obviously not as energetic as conventional cycling, but it's not a no-exercise option. It's a really great way of getting moderate-intensity activity.'[30]

Electric assistance is also helping to bring more activity back to the workplace. One of the fastest-changing areas of e-bikes is cargo bikes, where even a fairly small motor can help a rider carry loads into the hundreds of kilos. Such bikes are increasingly being used in some cities to replace vans for the so-called last mile of urban deliveries, from a city distribution point to people's addresses.

But these innovations are, again, often dependent on having sufficiently safe streets. It can be depressing to consider how far behind countries like the UK are lagging in terms of this. It is not just a matter of densely packed big cities. A few years ago I visited Odense, which while being Denmark's third-biggest city is a largely suburban place. Its generally spread-out population of about 200,000 people live mostly in houses, often with a garage, and generally with a car. But decades of work to build, at last count, around 350 miles of bike lanes and more than 120 cyclist-only bridges makes Odense a hugely welcoming place to cycle round. When I was there, city officials told me proudly that more than 80 per cent of children cycled to school, and – this was the statistic that most amazed me – the streets were now considered so safe that the official advice was that children should be perfectly able to cycle to school from the age of six. On their own.[31]

We in the UK can but dream of such movement-friendly urban landscapes, even if things might be about to shift at least slightly. One of the many things happening amid the coronavirus lockdown while I write this book is new government planning on how people can return to work but travel in socially distanced ways. With estimates that capacity on public transport could be cut by 90 per cent, and worries about gridlock if everyone drives, ministers have given local authorities new powers to carve out instant, temporary bike lanes using cones, and to widen pavements. The instruction has come: if you can walk or cycle to work, do so.

Could this spark a new active travel boom? Only time will tell, but the UK record on such matters is not a hopeful one. During our chat, Jan Gehl is politely pitying about my homeland, pointing out that not one UK city ever makes the various magazine lists of the world's most liveable places. 'I always say that Queen Elizabeth must have a traffic engineer's education to rule over such a country,' he jokes.

Just before I leave following our much-longer-than-scheduled talk, Gehl rummages in a folder and hands me a piece of paper. It is a street plan for a small housing development in the Danish town of Hobro, on the Jutland peninsula, for which his colleagues have been offering advice. Gehl shows me the many ways in which residents will be gently nudged towards activity. While there are roads circling the estate, and a couple within it, the houses are crisscrossed with a network of smaller, walking and cycling paths, making such rapid connections easy. Gehl then points out something not obvious from the plan: all the car parking for the development has been placed at one side, with public transport at another. The estate is on a hill, and if people want to reach their cars, they will have to climb up it. In contrast, the public transport is downhill. In their many efforts to invite people to be more active, Gehl's colleagues have even enlisted the assistance of gravity.

The hidden staircase

This crisis of designed inactivity is not, however, just about Gehl's life between buildings. It is also what we do inside them, particularly public ones like offices, shops and hotels. Among the most telling examples of a built environment biased against human movement is, as briefly mentioned in the opening chapter, the conspiracy of the hidden staircase.

I am a stair user by preference, in part because of a mild dislike of lifts. Sadly, this preference comes at a cost. Like most such people I could recount numerous examples of hunting vainly down hotel or office corridors for the telltale 'Fire exit' sign, not to mention the times I have accidentally triggered an alarm or found the stairwell doors only open from the outside, leaving me trapped in a windowless, fluorescent-lit concrete purgatory. When I first visited the London offices of the publishers of this book to discuss the idea, the route to the fire stairs in the 1970s office building was so complex that Fritha, who was to become my editor, had to not only guide me on the way up but lead me down again afterwards. It goes without saying that a set of gleaming lifts was immediately obvious when you first walked in.

The architecture of staircase use is a subject which might not immediately win you an audience at parties but is considerably more interesting than it might seem. I sought out experts to explain why stairwells are so often cramped, interior, unappealing and hard-to-find places. The obvious answer is that they are primarily also fire stairs, which to an extent dictates the design. It is possible to construct buildings with both fire stairs and another, more welcoming set of steps, but that adds to the costs.

Leon Rost, a New York–based partner at the Danish architectural firm Bjarke Ingels Group (BIG), points out another reason, particularly relevant for offices: such buildings tend to be designed so each floor can be rented out individually if required, and a spacious, obvious, front-of-house staircase on each level makes them less flexible, and thus potentially less lucrative.

Rost is fortunate enough to rarely have to worry about such things, given that his company specialises in bespoke, high-end buildings, often for the tech sector. He is leading the architectural team for the vast, still-under-construction new Google headquarters in California. Part of the brief for the futuristically named Googleplex in Mountain View, which will comprise about 200,000 square metres of office space, was to encourage as much physical movement by staff as possible.

As well as pedestrian walkways and bike lanes, the design emphasises the need for, in Rost's words, 'a natural way to entice people to move from building to building'. Trees and shade are a significant part of this, based on the idea known as biophilia, meaning that humans will instinctively seek contact with nature. With the new headquarters, Rost says, Google 'basically inherited a parking lot or suburban landscape, which is very un-enticing to go from building to building. If we can de-emphasise the space given over to vehicles and give more to nature, that alone gets people to move.'

The architects also hit on a slightly less subtle ruse to make sure Google's employees exert themselves at least a bit. The office has two storeys, with the work space almost all on the upper floor. On the ground level, connected by appealing, very obvi-ous courtyard-style staircases, are meeting rooms and cafés – as well as every single toilet, apart from accessible ones. If you need the loo, you use the stairs.

'Sundar loved that,' says Rost, referring to Sundar Pichai, the chief executive of Alphabet, Google's parent company. 'He was like, "We need to get these guys off their butts and moving around. Put everything on the ground floor except for water." Of course, if the stairs were locked inside of a concrete core, or if you had to find an elevator, that would be a drag, but we make those courtyards the best experience of the building.'[32]

Such design is important. When people become acclimatised over time to not using their body in the built environment, even when a flight of steps is very obviously there, it can go effectively unseen. One fascinating study tried to shift the physical decisions made by people by using nothing more than a reminder. A team of Glasgow University researchers put up signs saying, 'Stay Healthy, Save Time, Use the Stairs' at an underground rail station in the city centre, where passengers had the choice of an escalator or, right next to it, a thirty-step flight of stairs.

Observing passengers during the morning rush hour over a period of weeks, and excluding those with luggage or pushchairs, they found that a pre-sign stair usage of 8 per cent rose to more than 15 per cent during the three weeks that the signs were up. Even twelve weeks after the signs had been removed, stair use was significantly higher than the original figure, although on a gradual downward trend.[33]

It goes without saying that habitual stair use brings health benefits, and equally inevitably these have been proved via long-term mass studies. A 2019 paper using some of the decades of data from the Harvard Alumni Health Study, first developed by Ralph Paffenbarger, found that even after factoring out all other activity, habitual stair climbers (those who ascended thirty-five or more flights a week) had just 85 per cent of the mortality risk over the course of the study than those whose weekly average was ten or fewer.[34]

The big vision

Ideas about incorporating physical movement into architecture and planning have begun to move beyond staircases, occasionally in fairly startling ways. Amager Bakke, just east of central Copenhagen, is a huge waste-burning energy plant, designed as well by BIG. Also known as Copenhill, it is constructed with a huge sloping roof, on top of which is a dry skiing course as well as publicly open walking and hiking paths. When I travelled to visit Jan Gehl it had just opened and so I took one of Copenhagen's many public hire bikes and pedalled towards what, from a distance, looked like a hugely high-tech, angled, shiny shed, with a smoking chimney on top. I walked up the steep, rocky walking path to its 125-metre peak, from which padded skiers launched themselves down the angled, unnaturally green surface. Even with what are, by skiing standards, relatively cheap prices – an hour on the slope with all equipment is about £20 – no one would particularly mistake this for everyday activity. But as a statement as to what is possible it is quite something.

The most ambitious project in which Rost and BIG are involved, albeit so far only at the design stage, has been commissioned by Toyota, whose near-ninety years of producing reliable, affordable cars have played a fairly significant role in helping to create our inactive world.

The Japanese automaker has commissioned BIG to help design not just a human-friendly building, but an entire mini-metropolis. Toyota Woven City, to give the project its formal, slightly awkward name, is a planned 175-acre community to be built near Mount Fuji in Japan, which will not only be a home for its 2,000 or so residents but a test-bed for solutions to urban problems, including a move away from personal car use so residents can move around in different, often more active ways.

Only one in every three streets will be used by cars, with another third reserved for bikes and other types of, in the current buzzword, 'micro mobility', for example electric scooters, with the remainder of streets for pedestrian use only. The more human-oriented the street, the more nature will be included, as a way to tempt people out. Mundane logistics such as rubbish disposal and moving goods will be banished underground, an urban solution pioneered in Disneyland, with an emphasis on AI and robotics to do the work. All the cars, it should be mentioned, will be autonomous, testing out a form of transport on which several car makers, not only Toyota, are effectively betting the mortgage, but which has been found to be hugely difficult to integrate into real streets packed with smaller and sometimes arbitrarily moving objects such as people and bicycles.

Rost talks me through the plans with enthusiasm and a genuine passion for the ways they could make the urban realm more welcoming and inclusive. I am impressed, if not completely convinced. History might prove me wrong, but if towns and cities have a future in which physical activity becomes the norm, I'm not sure that technology, robotics and automation will be the primary reasons why.

A few years ago I had a long chat with a senior executive from Sidewalk Labs, a Google spinoff company which seeks to use tech to reimagine how cities could work in the future. We discussed how driverless cars – which at the time, as now, were confidently billed as being just around the corner from ubiquity – could affect active travel. While stressing that predictions were essentially guesswork, he conjured up one scenario in which autonomous cars sped people from distant suburbs to city centres, but with the last half mile or so, where people lived and worked, reserved for modes like cycling and walking. Again, I wasn't so sure. There is definitely an urban transport revolution coming, perhaps more quickly than most people realise, but it could go in several different ways.

The most feasible scenario, and certainly the one being most heavily pushed by governments in the UK and elsewhere, is a simple like-for-like replacement of petrol and diesel cars with electric ones. These would stop exhaust pollution, if not the spread of harmful particulates from tyre and brake wear. But that would be as far as the benefits went, not least on activity.

Chris Boardman is adamant it is not enough of a change. 'Electric cars are our biggest threat,' he tells me. 'And at the highest level of politics, people haven't heard it. Because these cars don't pollute, that's a good thing. But the unintended consequence is that you don't really get people to change anything. You won't touch health. You won't touch congestion, you won't touch road danger. I run an electric car. There's nothing wrong with an electric car. But it's not the bloody answer. It's part of the problem.'[35]

Another possibility, albeit in the slightly longer term, is the almost complete disappearance of all private cars from cities. But what will take their place? Will it be the hoped-for healthy mix of walking, cycling, public transport plus the occasional taxi or share ride? Or, if the technical challenges are finally met, could the newcomer be fleets of app-hailed driverless cars, an endlessly available, cheaper successor to Uber where people would expend even less energy than driving, dispensing with even the marginal exertion of pushing pedals and turning a steering wheel?

There is an alternative model to the slightly theme-park likes of Woven City. Vauban is a suburb in the south of Freiburg, a small and famously liveable city in the southwest of Germany. A former military base which for years was occupied only by squatters, Vauban was chosen in the late 1990s as the site for something of an experiment in sustainable, community-led living. Its design and ethos were set out by residents, who chose a layout of low-rise apartment blocks surrounded by green space. But the most radical idea was to dispense entirely with cars, even parking.

Under city laws, some parking had to be provided, but this was put all in one place, on the edge of the development, and is rarely used. Instead, the great majority of people rely on walking, bikes and an adjoining tram link into the city. The lack of cars, and particularly of parked cars, offers not just space but safety for everyday movement, including for children.

The photographs of Vauban looked so appealing that I planned a final research trip there for this book. My hope was to take my son, now nine, and see how it looked through his eyes. Then coronavirus intervened, scuppering travel of any sort. Luckily I was able to talk to Tim Gill, a British author, researcher and sometime government adviser who is an expert on mobility and play in children, and who had previously visited. 'I was there on a cold February afternoon, but the place was full of kids of different ages, with and without their parents, more or less occupying all of the available outdoor space,' Gill tells me. 'Of course, the space itself was well designed and had lots of playful features. But the first crucial step to really open up neighbourhoods and make built environments better for kids to be out and active is to take out cars.

'If you see the car as a consumer product, it's astonishing how many resources, both in terms of money but also physical space, we allow this consumer product to take up. Places like Vauban show what you can do if you just reconfigure neighbourhoods. The whole of the public realm then becomes a sociable, playful, welcoming space.'[36]

Movement for all

For all that I was perhaps a bit sceptical about BIG's Toyota Woven City concept, one theme it explores is hugely interesting. Among the reasons for the green, welcoming, car-free streets is to make the public realm more open to older people, and to those with disabilities. The former is particularly relevant given Japan has such a rapidly ageing population, with forecasts that around a third of all its population will be sixty-five or older within a decade from now.[37] The new Toyota community will, Rost tells me, be designed so older people 'feel invited to come outside'. He says: 'It's a continuation of the notion of accessibility. Right now it's considered to be a minimum requirement, almost like a tack-on, or a drag for architecture. But what if we think about it as a maximum – to make it extremely enticing and pleasurable, to draw people out.'

This is an important and often-neglected subject. Activity-thwarting design fails everyone, but it fails some more than others. Perhaps even less noticed than the divides of age and disability is the way so much of our public space discriminates against women and girls.

If I tally all the people I talked to in researching this book, around 40 per cent are women – a figure which could be higher. But then consider this chapter: you might not have noticed, but aside from the brief, in-passing mention of Rachel Aldred, every expert heard from so far has been male. An element is coincidence. But I'd argue it highlights a wider issue. The worlds of architecture and city planning have long had deserved reputations for being very male-dominated. In some areas this is changing, but there is still a long way to go. Even in a forward-thinking practice like BIG, of the seventeen partners, just two are women.[38]

Decades of male dominance have had inevitable repercussions for the built world, which has tended to be shaped, almost by default, for the needs of men. It is probably not a coincidence that in pretty much every country men and boys tend to be more active than women and girls. Both UK and global figures show that more women than men fail to meet minimum activity levels, usually by three or four percentage points. This gender gap is wider for children, particularly among adolescents.

Eva Kail possibly knows more about this divide than anyone.

A city planner in Vienna for almost thirty years, she has been a pioneer in pointing out the different ways that various groups of people navigate through a city, and their often competing needs. In 1991 she organised a pioneering and hugely popular photo exhibition about the female experience in the city's public space. The reaction to this was so positive that the city carried out a gender-based survey of transport use. It found that two thirds of car use, an area which dominated the city planning budget at the time, was done by men. The same proportion of walking trips involved women, but with hardly any consideration given to pedestrian welfare.

'That was really convincing for the politicians,' Kail tells me from Vienna. 'At the time, nobody spoke about pedestrian issues or about public space. Now public space is extremely hip.' The result was years of work in areas such as widening pavements to assist walking with a pushchair, and better lighting in pedestrian areas.

Much of this was instigated by a new *Frauenbüro*, or Women's Office, created in 1992 with Kail as its head. This also instigated wider city-planning efforts, seeking submissions from female architects. One early project was the *Frauen-Werk-Stadt*, or Women's Work City, a 350-unit housing complex in the north of the city. Designed to be welcoming and usable for women and families, much of this translated into assisting play and other types of activity, with safe areas for children to be outside, with clear sightlines from apartment windows. Similar projects have followed, the biggest of which is Aspern, an outer Vienna district where a family-friendly suburb of 20,000 people is being planned, and where all the streets will be named after women.

Kail is nonetheless still refreshingly outspoken about the attempts of her employer to redress the gender design balance: 'If you ask me, I think Vienna could do a lot more. If it comes to a conflict of interest – and in planning processes, it's all about the conflict of interest – it comes down to how much your perspective counts,' she says. 'You could call the gender strategy a bit of a good weather programme – if it doesn't hurt too much, maybe we can do it.'[39]

The often unconscious, in-built sexism of city planning is one of the areas highlighted by *Invisible Women*,[40] a fascinating and anger-inducing book by the British writer Caroline Criado-Perez, about the consequences of a world where the default design or decision is male. One example she highlights is the 2013 decision by Stockholm to change the order in which snowploughs cleared areas of the Swedish capital in winter. It had always started with the roads, and then the pavements and cycle paths. But as with 1990s Vienna, this disadvantaged the city's women, who are less likely to travel by car and more likely to walk or cycle. Criado-Perez notes in the book that in the UK, even during recent years of public spending costs, investment has been maintained in roads, on the apparent assumption this is the standard way to travel. And yet statistics show men drive on average twice as far a year as women.

One of the most pressing issues in modern public health is the way so many girls are lost from sports or other physical activities during adolescence. In the UK, teenage girls are about 10 per cent more likely than boys to do no sport at all, or to be inactive.[41] There are a variety of issues in play here but one of them is the design of urban recreational areas, which are almost all aimed at and used by – through inattention, if not actual design – predominantly boys.

To take one example very close to my life, my sister, her husband and their teenage daughter live in Frome, a town in Somerset. Over the past ten years or so the local council has built three outdoor activity or recreation facilities intended for older children, at a combined cost of £130,000: a skateboard park, a BMX track and a multi-use sports pitch. These are all used, almost entirely, by boys. Now the council plans to spend even more refurbishing the skate park. My sister is pushing the council to reconsider, pointing out that, so far, no sports facilities have been built with the needs and desires of girls in mind and that no equality assessments appear to have been carried out for any of these plans.

Thanks in large part to the efforts of Eva Kail and her colleagues, Vienna does think about how to make its parks and public sports facilities more welcoming to girls. Engagement at an early stage is the key, she says. Asked how cities can keep girls active, Kail tells me: 'It's very simple. You just have to talk to them, to watch them, and ask what they would like to do.'

Among ways to improve the gender mix, Kail says, is to avoid a single, fenced-in pitch, for example for football or basketball. 'We call them cages,' she says. 'This is really like the law of the jungle, because in this small cage there's only one playing field, and so the strongest take it over.' Kail and her planners instead developed a W-shaped area, with a series of separate, smaller spaces, so different groups can play at the same time. Some changes can be even more subtle, such as open entrances, rather than a gate which has to be opened.

'From watching girls it's clear that they are more timid, and also want to watch,' Kail says. 'So you need seating facilities, and then some quieter corners where they can also exist. This helps the less self-assertive groups. And if there are some open entrances then it's easier for the weaker groups to come in. All these open-air playgrounds are much more designed for boys' interests.'

In terms of particular sports, Kail says, girls in Vienna have tended to enjoy volleyball or using slacklines. 'These are things where you have separation, where you don't have close contact with the enemy,' she explains. 'This is what girls really like. And for them it's also about meetings and social life, to sit together and chat in small groups, in a half-protected position so you can have an overview of what's going on, but you also feel a bit sheltered.'

And skate parks, the supposedly gender-neutral choice of Frome and so many other UK towns and cities? Kail views them as a symbol of how far this consideration of gender and activity still has to go. 'We are still a bit at the beginning of this discussion,' she says. 'Skate parks are very hip now, and they take up a lot of public space, but again it's a very male interest, and a very hard sport. Girls can be so modest sometimes, and it would be great if they could be given more space and more independence.'

Next steps:

For most people, active travel is the biggest activity gain there is. Think about how you get around. Could you replace some shorter car trips with walking or cycling? Could you ride to and from your job or place of study? There are far too many potential tips for enjoyable cycling to list here, so maybe ask friends or colleagues who already cycle. But one idea is to try to use a quieter, back-street route. There are plenty of phone apps which will plan these and, if you attach your phone to the handlebars, can give step-by-step directions.

6

Being Slim Isn't Enough: Why Inactivity and Obesity are Different

When Tom Watson first decided to become more active as part of efforts to turn around a lifestyle he feared was on course to kill him, he started with the very basics. The then-Labour MP, who spent four years as deputy leader of his party, had been overweight since his twenties. By now he was fifty and clinically obese, weighing somewhere near 22 stone, or 140 kilos. One early part of this new regime, Watson tells me, involved trying to walk a bit more, something he admits was not exactly a long-standing habit. 'Before, a five-minute walk would have been too much,' he says. 'I would have felt it was a waste of time – why walk somewhere when a cab can get you there marginally quicker? I started with a target of 5,000 steps a day, which for me was quite a challenge. At first, if I walked even half that, like from parliament to my flat, I'd feel a little light-headed from the exertion.'[1]

When I speak to Watson it is two and a half years on from

that time, and he is around eight stone (50kg) lighter, having had to, along the way, replace more or less his entire wardrobe of clothes. We speak on the phone – even after quitting parliament he is permanently busy – and as we chat he is striding between one engagement near Covent Garden in London towards another in Whitechapel, just over two miles to the east.

Watson says he now aims for 12,500 steps a day, 'and I probably get way over that five out of seven days'. The previous evening, after dinner with a friend in north London, he spent more than an hour walking to his flat, just south of the Thames. 'The city opens up to you when you walk around it,' Watson says. 'Now a walk is an absolute joy. What a privilege it is to be able to find an hour to be able to do it. It's a completely different relationship with movement that I have.'

The trigger for Watson's decision to change his life, as he recounts in *Downsizing*,[2] his very readable and well-researched autobiography-meets-treatise on the slimming process, came a few years earlier at a party. A guest he had never met before, a doctor, told Watson that given his weight and extent of stomach fat, along with sweaty skin and frequent trips to the toilet, he most likely had undiagnosed type 2 diabetes. This turned out to be correct, although with the subsequent weight loss and increase in activity, Watson's diabetes is now in complete remission. Before he started to transform his lifestyle, Watson tells me, he began with 'pretty powerful periods of self-reflection'. He says: 'I literally thought that if I didn't change I would die. That took time to sink in, to realise the magnitude of that. And then I just thought, "Okay, you don't want to die, how do you get out of it?"'

Watson's eventual answer to this self-posed question gets to the heart of the complex and intertwined relationship between excess weight and inactivity, which this chapter examines. As well as gradually becoming more active, he completely reshaped his diet, not just the amount he ate but the types of food. For Watson, this meant cutting out all forms of sugars and processed carbohydrates and adopting the so-called keto diet, which instead involves considerable fat intake. While proponents argue this can both help lose weight and improve the body's relationship with insulin, at the centre of type 2 diabetes, some nutritionists urge caution. It is a vexed issue, and I'm not about to start offering specific advice on diets. But the type of food regime Watson decided to adopt is, to an extent, irrelevant. The wider point is that physical activity and losing weight are by no means the same thing. Yes, regular physical exertion is hugely helpful in maintaining a healthy weight and can assist with gradual weight loss. But, as we'll see later, barring a pretty extreme and virtually all-day exercise programme, movement alone is not enough to prompt the sort of physical transformation experienced by Watson. You also need a reduction in caloric intake, involving a healthy mix of foods.

This brings us to another key point, perhaps the most important in this chapter: even weight loss is to an extent a secondary issue, and certainly in health terms. This can sound an anomalous, even heretical thing to say in our era of – entirely justified – worries about the global public health crisis caused by obesity. And it is not to suggest that losing weight is irrelevant. All things being equal, someone of what doctors would term a normal weight has better average health outcomes than someone who is overweight, particularly so if the excess weight moves into clinical obesity.

But this is not the only calculation in play. To begin with, as we'll see in a minute, weight, as judged by the standard metric of body mass index (BMI), is not the only gauge, with research increasingly showing that other measurements such as waist size and the location of body fat can be equally, if not more, relevant for health. Also, study after study has shown that someone who is active generally receives health benefits even if they are overweight, though again this effect tends to diminish with serious obesity. Finally – and this is where things get perhaps the most controversial – some research suggests that, overall, it could be better for your health outcomes to be regularly physically active and have some excess weight than it is to be slim and immobile.

While this 'fat and fit' narrative is still challenged by some academics, it is undoubtedly true that if someone is overweight it is just as important for them to be active as it is for anyone else, perhaps even more so. However, becoming active can be particularly challenging for people who start the process obese. Part of this can be the sheer effect of the weight, as Tom Watson recalls: 'Imagine carrying eight stone in a rucksack. It's a lot more tiring. And your physical movement is restricted.' There are other practical obstacles for heavier people seeking to be active. For example, some bicycles have recommended weight limits of 120kg, which would have excluded Watson. The same is true for many home running treadmills.

But perhaps the greatest issue is stigma. Obesity is a hugely complicated issue, as much so as inactivity, and is shaped by all sorts of factors which are beyond the control of any individual, especially someone living in more deprived circumstances. This is another hugely broad and complex subject, going into psychology as well as the lived environment, and also beyond the scope of this book. But the general principle must be noted. To take one key example, we live in an era in which an increasing amount of the foodstuffs on offer are highly processed and often laden with ingredients like high-fructose corn syrup. They are made by corporate giants who ensure the products are prominently displayed on supermarket shelves and heavily marketed to households.

Tom Watson says he was formerly a 'sugar addict', and is scathing about the malign power of the food industry in shaping what people eat: 'I now go into supermarkets and there are whole aisles of just zero-nutrition, highly calorific, highly industrialised, processed foods. Whereas before I would literally salivate looking at the packets, now they're just lost to me. You really realise the very deeply ingrained axiomatic responses we have to certain foods.'

Watson's book describes how, as a politician, he experienced the influence of 'Big Sugar' in shaping government decisions. This resonated with me – even as a journalist I've seen how this can work. A couple of years ago, while researching a news story connected to lobbying efforts by food corporations, I received a letter from the very expensive lawyers representing one of the companies, warning of dire consequences should we publish the piece. I'm lucky enough to work for a newspaper with very good lawyers of our own, who could quickly see the threat was baseless. But as a vignette it demonstrates the forces at work.

Scientists have examined other impacts of this obesogenic foodscape, as they describe it, on people's diets. One alarming study of an area of Cambridgeshire in the UK measured the number of takeaway outlets within a mile radius of people's homes and workplaces, and on their commutes. Aside from the sheer amount – the average person was exposed to just over nine outlets at home and on their commute, and almost fourteen at work – it found that of the 5,000-plus people surveyed, those in the top 25 per cent group whose environment was most saturated with takeaway outlets were more than twice as likely to be obese compared to those in the bottom 25 per cent.[3] That research was from 2014, before the era of ubiquitous, app-based food ordering services. Now, you don't even need to leave the house to face this obesogenic world; it's right there in your pocket.

And yet societal prejudice towards excess weight is rife, prompting feelings of shame and humiliation which can become particularly intense when physical exertion is involved. A US study about overweight people who went to gyms found those who were obese in particular felt particular stigma, which affected their motivation. 'Worrying that other people will laugh at me or judge me,' one person wrote when asked to explain why they were wary about going. 'Fearing that I will break or damage equipment because of my weight,' said another.[4]

Tom Watson recalls how he would habitually stigmatise himself for three decades: 'I used to describe myself as the hardest-working laziest person I knew. I self-identified as overweight and lazy and slothful because of all the caricatures, but there was the contradiction of working eighteen hours a day, seven days a week. I couldn't work it out. There's this sort of binary idea about health and weight loss and wellbeing, that it's down to the individual. And yes, it is ultimately about very deeply personal decisions about what you put in yourself and how you expend energy, but the system is stacked against you.'

Given the overwhelmingly strong evidence that increased activity helps someone's health more or less whatever their weight, such attitudes are deeply alarming. Dr Robert Ross, from Queen's University in Ontario, Canada, is one of the world's leading researchers on the interaction between excess weight and activity. While Ross stresses his job does not officially cover behavioural science, he recognises the attitudes many overweight and obese people face, particularly when they begin to become active. 'Sometimes, obesity in some people's eyes is the last justifiable prejudice,' Ross tells me. 'People look at someone who is overweight or obese and automatically assume "lazy", "inconsiderate" and things like that. And for many if not most, nothing could be farther from the truth. If we want people that are overweight and obese to engage in physical activity and to consume a balanced, healthful diet, we have to make those healthy choices easier choices. It's not a question of being lazy, it's a question of just how difficult it is in today's environment to do it.'

It is, Ross says, a prejudice which is particularly directed at women: 'This is my opinion, but I do believe there's a gender difference. For a male to have a little bit of an expanded waist-line, if he has grey hair and smoked a cigar, you could be a CEO of a company. But when a woman has the expanded waistline we say things like "lazy", and we say things like "not pretty", and this is such a shame. We've seen that in our own research programmes.'[5]

More than one metric

It's worth mentioning what is meant by BMI, the standard measure for excess weight. It is your weight in kilograms divided by the square of your height in metres, and there are numerous websites which calculate this for you, as well as converting non-metric measurements. There is a much-used guide for BMI which states that if yours is below 18.5 you are classed as underweight, with anything from 18.5 to 25 seen as healthy. From 25 and above, we are in the realm of excess weight, but this is divided into four sections, with varying health risks for each. At 25 to 30 people are classified as overweight, or 'pre-obese'. There are then three levels of obesity: BMIs of 30 to 35, 35 to 40, and 40 and above, with the last one sometimes labelled 'extreme' or 'severe' obesity.

An important point must be stressed here: while this is seen as the 'standard' set of measures, it is based on white European ethnicity, and the danger levels can vary for people of other heritage. The biggest potential impact is for people from an Asian background, whether South Asian or East Asian, where health concerns appear to set in at slightly lower BMIs. For example, one huge long-term US study into women and the prevalence of type 2 diabetes found that at the same BMI levels, women from Asian backgrounds had more than twice the risk of developing diabetes over the twenty-year course than their white peers. Hispanic and African-American women also had a slightly higher risk, though not to the same extent.[6] The reasons for this difference are not fully understood, although one factor is believed to be that Asian people, particularly those of South Asian descent, can have up to 5 per cent more body fat than someone of the same BMI from a European background.[7] The World Health Organization (WHO) thus now recommends that for Asian people, the threshold for being overweight should be a BMI of 23 rather than 25, with obesity starting at 27.5, and not 30.[8]

Another caveat to mention here is that the theories about any benefits of activity potentially exceeding the perils of weight are only really argued in the lower categories. If your BMI is 40, that means even an average-height UK man would weigh something over 120kg, or nearly 19 stone. That is not a healthy weight in the long term. For any long-term benefit someone of this BMI would need to lose weight as well as become more active.

What is clear is that excess weight is an increasingly significant, worldwide problem, with an extent that is almost shocking to comprehend. In England, just under two thirds of adults have an excessively high BMI. Of these, an estimated 35 per cent are overweight (a BMI between 25 and 30) and another 28 per cent are classified as obese.[9] Statistics are collected separately by each UK nation, and England is not the worst – in Scotland the figures are 40 per cent of people overweight and 29 per cent obese.[10]

This situation varies by age and is more common in men. Of English men aged between fifty-five and sixty-four, more than 80 per cent are overweight or obese.[11] There is also a significant correlation with economic and social hardship, particularly for women. In the English districts classified as being in the most deprived fifth of the total, 35 per cent of men and 37 per cent of women are obese. In the best-off category, the figures fall to 20 per cent and 21 per cent.[12] Excess weight might not be explicitly a disease of poverty, as with the rheumatic heart disease seen by Jerry Morris in Chapter 3, but the evidence is very clear that to characterise it as a condition dictated by willpower, let alone greed or indolence, is utterly mistaken, and does nothing to make the situation any better.

It is also increasingly a condition of childhood. Currently, 28 per cent of English children (those aged two to fifteen) are overweight or obese, of whom 15 per cent are classified as obese.[13] Worldwide, things are generally no better, although the extent of excess weight does still vary massively between nations. The most recent estimates by WHO, for 2016, say that globally, 39 per cent of adults are overweight or obese, with about 13 per cent classified as obese. The prevalence of obesity around the world nearly tripled between 1975 and 2016, the organisation says. The rise in excess weight for children and adolescents has been even more dramatic. While in 1975, just 4 per cent of those aged five to nineteen had excess weight, with 1 per cent obese, the equivalent 2016 figures were 18 per cent and 7 per cent.[14]

In a 2016 speech on the crisis, the WHO's then-director general, Dr Margaret Chan, noted that in just a few decades the world had 'moved from a nutrition profile in which the prevalence of underweight was more than double that of obesity, to the current situation in which more people worldwide are obese than underweight'. The shift towards what she termed population-wide obesity was, Chan said, 'a slow-motion disaster'.[15]

One study illustrates the still considerable differences in obesity between different parts of the world. The research, published in 2014 in *The Lancet*, showed that at least 50 per cent of men were now classified as obese – not just overweight – in Tonga, with the same for women in Kuwait, Kiribati, Micronesia, Libya, Qatar, Tonga and Samoa. For children and teenagers, obesity levels varied from over 30 per cent for girls in Kiribati, Samoa and Micronesia to less than 2 per cent in countries like Bangladesh, Cambodia and Laos. The vast, 140-strong authorial team noted gloomily that they had 'found no countries where there have been significant declines over the last 33 years'.

They said: 'This raises the question as to whether many or most countries are on a trajectory to reach the high levels of obesity observed in countries such as Tonga or Kuwait.' The one slightly hopeful note they added was the observation that, given rates of increase seem to be slowing in some developed countries, especially among younger people, the epidemic might have peaked in a few places.[16]

Excess weight is a particular worry in countries which have seen rapid economic development in recent decades, notably China. The most recent estimates say 46 per cent of Chinese adults and 15 per cent of children are overweight or obese.[17] China might have the greatest absolute number of overweight people, but India is not so far behind, with one 2019 study finding that suddenly inactive lifestyles and the arrival of high-calorie foods meant anything up to a third of Indian adults were classified as obese.[18]

All of this does, of course, come at a significant economic cost, both to health systems and more widely. NHS figures say that in England alone, 710,000 people every year are admitted to hospital with obesity cited as a primary or secondary cause.[19] This is connected to dozens of medical problems, ranging from arthritis to heart disease or pneumonia, as well as the effects of excess weight on pregnant women and foetal health. Calculating an overall economic cost is hugely difficult, but one study by the London-based World Obesity Forum, which gathers scientific expertise on the subject, estimated that by 2025 the total global bill connected to obesity would be around £950 billion.[20]

The association of excess weight with generally poorer health outcomes has been highlighted anew by the coronavirus pandemic. To reiterate, this book is being written during the period of its peak in the UK, and many of the public health lessons are only emerging. But one repeated feature of studies both in China and Europe has been the greater probability of obese patients to require hospital treatment for the Covid-19 virus, and also to die.

The energy balance

How did the world get to this point? The answer in its broadest terms was expressed with great eloquence more than sixty years ago by one of the first experts to warn about the then-nascent obesity crisis. Jean Mayer, a French-American nutritionist who advised three US presidents on the subject, is yet another of the extraordinary but now virtually forgotten figures to crop up in this book. Mayer was a genuine pioneer in research on nutrition, encompassing an era of transition in which he could simultaneously warn about the need for extra food assistance for America's poor, and about the consequences for others who were well fed but increasingly inactive.

Like Jerry Morris, Mayer's life story was astounding enough on its own. Born in Paris in 1920, he was captured by the invading Germans in 1940 while fighting as an artillery lieutenant, later escaping from a prisoner of war camp. Over the rest of the war Mayer worked for the French underground and then as a British agent, fought with Free French and then Allied forces in North Africa and Europe, and served on General Charles de Gaulle's staff in London, eventually receiving fourteen decorations, including the Croix de Guerre and the Resistance Medal.

After the war he married an American woman and took a postgraduate course at Yale, becoming a nutritionist, then a noted expert on how to tackle famines overseas. But he also researched the importance of balancing food intake with activity levels as a way to prevent obesity, a particularly far-sighted approach in a time when, as one of Mayer's colleagues later put it, 'obesity in humans was seen as the result of some sort of character defect'.[21] His research discovered that while people tend to compensate for increased exertion by eating more food, the converse is not true: when someone becomes less active, their appetite does not normally diminish to match it. This creates what is technically known as a 'continued positive energy balance' – consistently eating more calories than you expend – and thus excess weight.

Noting the fact that even 1950s Americans were moving far less than those a generation before, Mayer warned in 1955 that many of them faced a dilemma, given that their bodies were seemingly not able to adjust to being satiated with less food.

'In many cases, adaptation to modern conditions without development of obesity implies that the person will have to either step up his activity or endure mild or acute hunger all his life,' he wrote in The Physiological Basis of Obesity and Leanness. 'If the first alternative, stepping up activity, is difficult, it is well remembered that the second alternative, lifetime hunger, is so much more difficult that to rely on it for weight control in cases of sedentary overweight can only continue the fiascos of the past.'[22]

The subsequent decades have proved Mayer correct. While eating a relatively moderate, balanced diet is of course essential for maintaining a healthy weight, simply imploring people to eat a bit less doesn't really solve anything. Their activity levels also need to step up. And as we have seen, even if a minority of people are throwing themselves into regular, vigorous, organised exercise, the everyday world has changed so much that overall activity has, on average, diminished.

This is perhaps the one certainty of the intake/output debate when it comes to excess weight at population-wide levels. Curiously, while it is often assumed that people today eat consistently more calories than earlier generations, this is up for some debate, and in part depends on who you ask. One study based on US census data calculated that the average American in 2010 consumed 2,481 calories per day, 20 per cent more than their peers in 1970, with the make-up of food also considerably changed, including less sugar but considerably more high-fructose corn syrup.[23] In contrast, a study of food consumption in England between 1980 and 2013 calculated that total intake had actually fallen, despite a shift from calories from home-cooked meals towards those in restaurant food, takeaways, drinks and snacks. The researchers suggested that the increase in spending on food caused by more eating out had led in part to an assumption that more was being eaten.[24]

Yet another complication is that basing any assessment on how much people say they eat is a perilous business. One UK government statistical study from 2018, which surveyed what people said they ate and then accurately measured the actual calories consumed, found that people tended to wildly underestimate. Men declared an average daily intake of 2,033 calories, and women 1,584 calories, both well under the recommended intake of 2,500 and 2,000 calories. But the researchers found the actual average was 3,119 calories a day for men, and 2,393 for women.[25]

To an extent, such debates are beside the point. For as long as so many people are living less actively, unless their food intake is reduced to compensate, over time their weight will increase. Time is a key factor here. A continued positive energy balance does not need to be very great at all to prompt a significant difference in weight, if maintained over the months and years. According to calculations in a book chapter on obesity co-authored by Robert Ross, someone who is just ten calories a day above what is termed their 'weight maintenance energy requirement' will gain about half a kilo a year, which is in fact the current average increase for middle-aged Americans.[26]

Ten calories, as you can imagine, is very, very little food, perhaps a bite of a chocolate bar, or a part-teaspoon of mayonnaise. More positively, to burn up those ten calories in activity is a matter of just a very brief walk. And as Jean Mayer pointed out at the beginning of the obesity crisis, as a way of reorganising one's life, being more active can often be more straightforward than eating less.

Numerous studies have demonstrated Mayer's maxim that the body tends not to limit its appetite when daily movement is reduced. One particularly thorough Scottish project involved taking six healthy if generally inactive men in their early twenties and essentially treating them as laboratory rodents for two seven-day periods. They spent each week in what is known as a 'whole body calorimeter', a sealed-off, space age–looking pod inside of which the oxygen they consumed and the carbon dioxide they produced could be measured, which allowed an accurate calculation of their total energy expenditure. On both weeks, the volunteers were able to eat however much food they wanted at three set meal times, chosen from a menu. The food was delivered via an airtight hatch, a process which must presumably have increased the lab rat ambience all the more.

The difference between the weeks was that in one of them, each volunteer was instructed to be inactive, limited to a total daily exertion of just 1.4 of their basal metabolic rate (BMR), or resting state. If you remember this from Chapter 2, a figure of 1.4 puts someone in the more-or-less completely sedentary category, only slightly above a patient in a hospital bed. On the other week – the order of the weeks was randomly chosen and the subjects were not told the purpose of the experiment – the volunteers were instructed to carry out three exercise bike sessions a day in their sealed pods, pushing their total daily energy expenditure to 1.8 times BMR, the sort of figure you might see in a manual job.

Although there was, as you would expect, considerable difference between the energy expended in the active and sedentary weeks, the researchers found that food intake was broadly similar for both. The volunteers did consume slightly more calories during the active phase, but this was due to a greater intake of caloric fluids like soft drinks. There was also, the academics noted, 'no tendency for energy intake to drop as the sedentary regimen progressed'.

The extent of excess eating during the artificially immobile week was striking. The average combined excess energy balance for the test subjects over the sedentary seven days was just over 3,600 calories, sufficient for a massive 25kg in weight gain if maintained over a year. Interestingly, the experiment found that the subjects also ate slightly more than they needed during the active period, albeit only slightly, a result which might, of course, simply demonstrate the habit of many young men to eat as much food as they can if it is available without effort or cost.[27]

This imbalance between intake and exertion is a fascinating area, and can vary greatly between different people. Another study put a group of men and women through three progressively more intense exercise regimes over a sixteen-day period using stationary bikes or treadmills, again comparing their energy output and food intake. This showed two things. One was the body's general tendency not to fully account for extra exertion – on average the test subjects only made up 30 per cent of the increased energy they expended in additional food intake. The other was that this was by no means a uniform effect. About half the group ate more, and the others didn't.[28]

This shows the split between what researchers call 'compensators' and 'non-compensators'. While I don't wish to create any new artificial divisions in an already atomised world, in much the same way as you can divide people into, say, those who believe it's acceptable to recline an airline seat on a short-haul flight and those who argue that this should be punishable by prison, the idea of compensators and non-compensators does resonate very strongly. I firmly fall into the former camp, as someone who both enjoys staying active but also does so as a way to enjoy more of the foods I love, in the belief it will not affect my body composition (as you will see later, this has not proved an infallible maxim). It's not that I think people who feel differently are wrong, just that they appear to be speaking a slightly different physical language.

Worshipping the scales

All these studies point fundamentally towards the same conclusion. Irrespective of modern dietary changes, the much-proved reduction in overall average physical activity around the world plays a very significant role in the parallel crisis of obesity. The health risks of obesity cross over significantly with those of inactivity, but are not precisely the same, both in terms of scope and intensity.

In the previously mentioned textbook chapter about obesity co-authored by Robert Ross, there is an eloquent chart citing various health conditions associated with excess weight, with between one and four upward-pointing arrows showing the degree of risk associated with obesity. One arrow indicates an increased risk of 25 per cent–50 per cent; two means a 200 per cent increase; three arrows is around 350 per cent; while four stands for more than 400 per cent additional risk. The four-arrow warning is given to type 2 diabetes, while three arrows is next to pulmonary embolism (a blood clot in the lungs), arthritis and chronic back pain. The two-arrow designation is given to coronary artery disease, high blood pressure, kidney and pancreatic cancers and gallbladder disease. In the final, one-arrow group, come asthma, colorectal cancer, breast cancer in older women and the big ones – stroke, heart failure and early death.[29] This is, of course, in part dependent on the extent of weight, with numerous studies showing that once BMI hits around 30, or especially 40 (the threshold of severe obesity), the risks multiply.

There is also the parallel issue of morbidity – someone's ability to live independently and in good health. One US study which measured the changing health outcomes from obesity over fifteen years noted that while death rates had actually fallen, this could be largely because of improved medical care, and that the amount of impairment and disability caused by excess weight was both increasing and taking effect in people from an ever-younger age.[30]

There is another big subject to consider with the health risks of weight: it depends where the weight is. Increasing amounts of research have shown the particular importance of fat around the waist. Visceral, or intra-abdominal fat, makes up just 10 per cent or so of your body's total fat content (the rest is subcutaneous fat, the layer just below the skin), but is the focus of many health worries. These are fat cells in the visceral peritoneum, the inner layer of a membrane wrapped around internal organs like the liver and stomach. Quite why visceral fat is so risky is not completely understood. One idea, known as portal theory,[31] argues that visceral fat transmits substances which can promote inflammation to the liver via the portal vein. This can cause insulin resistance, as well as liver steatosis, otherwise known as non-alcoholic fatty liver, which has a series of potential health consequences of its own. Another idea is based around visceral fat's role in releasing cytokines, molecules which transmit signals to cells and can also provoke inflammation.

This is why obesity experts increasingly use measures such as waist size, or a waist-to-height ratio, as a gauge of the potential health risks of excess weight, rather than BMI alone. BMI can be a blunt tool, not least as it doesn't distinguish between muscle and fat. Thus, as some rugby players will tell you at great length, it is possible for a hugely fit and very built-up professional athlete to have a BMI above 25, officially making them overweight.

Robert Ross is the lead author of a statement released in 2020 by more than a dozen experts in the field that advises governments and medical practitioners to focus less on BMI and more on waist size. 'Decreases in waist circumference are a critically important treatment target for reducing adverse health risks for both men and women,' it says. The paper warns that while BMI measurements are starting to plateau in some countries, waist circumference figures appear to still be on the increase, potentially masking the extent of the obesity-related health crisis.[32]

Ross told me that he is a firm believer in the value of waist size as a guide to weight-related health: 'Our evidence would clearly suggest that you can reduce your waist circumference without substantial reductions in body weight. Now, if you're losing weight, I've never seen anybody gain in the waist. I, myself, use my pant size. I haven't been on a scale in, seriously, thirty years. I've got no idea. My pants tell me how I'm doing.' BMI remains a useful measure, he stresses, just ideally not used on its own: 'I'm not one that promotes drop-kicking BMI into the Atlantic Ocean. If you want to stratify an adult's obesity-related health risk, then measure both.'[33]

Waist circumference is a particularly important measure in the rise of type 2 diabetes, which is the condition that most closely connects inactivity and obesity, and forms perhaps the greatest part of the resultant global public health crisis. Estimates suggest almost one in ten of the world's population is living with diabetes, the vast majority of them the type 2 variant and with almost half of them, as happened with Tom Watson, doing so with the condition undiagnosed. Taking into account undiagnosed cases, anything up to 4 million Britons have it.[34] And the risk from excess weight is proved beyond doubt. The mechanism is complex and still not fully understood, as we saw in Chapter 2, but seems driven by the increased presence of cytokines and other substances associated with inflammation, which can provoke insulin resistance.

Again, much of this is connected to visceral fat, hence the importance of waist size – something shown in numerous stud-ies. One major European research project which tracked more than 25,000 adults over an average of nine years found that each centimetre increase in waist size brought an 8 per cent increase in the risk of diabetes. Strikingly, the researcher found that men and women with a normal BMI of below 25 but an unhealthy waist circumference had a 3.6 times increased risk of developing the condition, more than the 2.6 increase faced by those with a BMI of between 25 and 30 but a healthy waist size.[35]

There is also strong evidence about the more general health risks of an increased waist size. One 2014 meta-study, which pooled data from more than 650,000 adults of all ages over an average of nine years, found that after factoring out other circumstances, a higher waist circumference was linked with a greater risk of death at every level of BMI, from 20 to 50. This meant, the authors noted, that even in people of what is seen as a normal weight, waist size should be monitored as a potential health risk.[36]

Another issue with a fixation on BMI is that, as we shall see soon, losing weight via increased activity can be a long, arduous and often dispiriting process. But even if someone's BMI remains stubbornly consistent, their health could still be improving, with a decrease in waist circumference often indicating this. 'Anecdotally we hear that all the time,' Robert Ross says. 'Someone will come up and say, "Gee, Dr Ross, I'm not losing the weight that I wanted to despite my good eating habits and physical activity. But interestingly enough, this dress fits a lot better, or my pants fit a lot better. It's just the darned bathroom scale." I joke that Moses came down the mountain with two tablets and a bathroom scale. We worship that thing. Some people get on that scale and if it doesn't say what they want, they feel poorly about themselves, despite engaging in healthy behaviours. And that's so unfortunate, truly a missed opportunity.'

So what is a healthy waist size? As with BMI, this is to an extent approximate, and also like BMI it varies across ethnic groups. But for white adults, the metric first devised in 1995 by the pleasingly named Professor Mike Lean of Glasgow University, and still seen as the standard, suggests that, irrespective of your height or BMI, a waist size of more than 37 inches (94cm) in men and 31.5 inches (80cm) in women is potentially unhealthy and should be reduced.[37] Once you get above 40 inches (102cm) for men and 34.5 inches (88cm) for women, NHS guidance says you are 'at very high risk of some serious health conditions and should see a GP'.[38] The figures are again slightly less for people of South or East Asian background, with the health risks seen as starting at 35.5 inches (90cm) in men and 31.5 inches (80cm) in women.

As Robert Ross noted, the relevance of waist size to activity is that people tend to see the effects much more quickly than they do with BMI. When it comes to weight loss, many are surprised to learn quite how much exertion is needed to achieve this, without a parallel programme of diet control, or even how much is recommended if your only goal is to stay roughly the same weight. Yes, the government-recommended level of at least 150 minutes a week of moderate activity or equivalent will provide almost endless health benefits. But weight loss – and perhaps even weight maintenance – will probably not be among them.

A statement released almost twenty years ago by a series of leading experts in the field of activity and weight laid out what is generally seen as the consensus view: even to remain the same weight, people need to aim for at least forty-five to sixty minutes of moderate exertion a day, every day. If someone was obese and had slimmed down, an even greater amount of movement is needed to stay slim – anything from sixty to ninety minutes a day.[39]

So how much activity is required to lose significant amounts of weight, without a parallel change in diet? To answer this we must turn to perhaps the most fascinating and also one of the more alarming studies ever carried out in the field of physical activity research. It took place in Bulgaria in 1982, and the resulting full academic paper – nowadays so rare I had to order a copy from the British Library – certainly has a very Eastern Bloc feel to it.

Led by the slightly sinister-sounding Institute of Hygiene and Occupational Health in Sofia, it followed the fortunes of thirty-two women who came from what was described as 'a sanatorium for obese patients'. Over the 45-day course of the study the women lost an impressive average of 12.4kg, about one eighth of their body weight, at the same time seeing their body fat proportion fall from 38 per cent to 31 per cent. This happened while they ate an average of 2,780 calories per day, well over the amount normally needed to maintain weight, let alone lose so much.

How did they do it? As you read further down the study it begins to make sense. Every day they were put through an exercise programme lasting about ten hours. The daily group regime for the women – who are described as 'volunteers', although I have my doubts – comprised this: fifteen minutes of gymnastics; an hour of 'standing exercises'; an hour of gymnastics using apparatus; two hours of 'walks and long-distance races'; three hours of 'sports and athletic games'; and finally an hour of what is described, cryptically and disconcertingly, as 'therapeutic dances'. In addition, the women did individual exercises including swimming, tennis, and more 'long-distance races'. If that was not enough to break their spirit, there was also a weekly 'walking tour' of an initial 20km, a distance which increased by 5km every week.

The result, the study boasts, was 'statistically significant decrease in weight and percentage of body fat'. This is perhaps not surprising, given it also found that the participants expended an average of 3,700 calories per day.[40] As a comparison, a 2019 study of footballers in the Dutch premier league, the *Eredivisie*, discovered their average daily physical exertion was a mere 3,300 calories.[41] As a regime, this punishing exercise programme definitely shed the weight. But it is perhaps not so straightforward, let alone appealing, to transfer into everyday life.

The right message

The message thus seems fairly clear. Unless you are able to clear your diary for the foreseeable future to incorporate a pretty extreme activity regime, should your goal be to lose a lot of weight then you will need to address your diet as well as physical movement. Again, I'm not about to get into how weight loss can best be achieved, but it is worth stressing that it tends to be pretty challenging, as is maintaining the loss. Numerous studies have examined the issue of weight recidivism, and the consensus seems to be that over a period of year or so, the majority of dieters regain some or all of what they lost. Much of this seems to be the body's innate resistance, built up over millennia of coping with food lack rather than excess, to oppose repeated negative energy balances, fighting back with metabolic changes, for example to boost the appetite.

Tom Watson's book is a useful chronicle of the sheer effort required to shed significant amounts of weight in a fairly brief time. A self-professed borderline obsessional character, Watson read endless scientific studies on diets, completely cut out sugars, and bought a set of electronic scales which he synchronised with his mobile phone to get the satisfaction, as he put it, of 'watching the graph going down over time'. As well as completely reshaping what he ate, his activity regime included not just walking, but increasing amounts of cycling, and visits to a series of gyms. For one particularly rigorous period he lifted weights three days a week in what he calls 'an extraordinarily expensive' gym. 'The results were amazing,' he says. 'I described it as getting a body I didn't deserve in a gym I couldn't afford. But for those two months the whole world revolved around the gym and nutrition in the gym. And that wasn't my goal.'

Watson's gym regime also highlights the increasing focus on weights-based activity, as well as aerobic exertion, as a way to combat excess weight, even though the results seem to happen more on reducing waist size and body fat percentage rather than lowering BMI. There is another potential benefit. As some studies have noted, aerobic exercise like running or cycling, even brisk walking, can be difficult for people who are overweight or obese, whereas lifting weights might appear more feasible.

Some form of lifting weights, whether in a gym or as part of everyday life, also appears especially important in the management of type 2 diabetes, with numerous studies noting that the effects can be as beneficial as those of aerobic activity. Much of this appears to be linked to the importance of our mass of skeletal muscle in bodily health. It is in skeletal muscle where the bulk of glucose uptake after meals takes place, and insulin resistance here appears to be one of the very beginning elements of type 2 diabetes. Working your muscles is also linked to better functioning mitochondria, and the improved processing of fats, both of which reduce the risk of diabetes.

All this is useful, but still leaves someone who is overweight, whether gauged by BMI, waist size or both, in roughly the same place as before. So, assuming they do not have the time, resources and focus to attempt a Tom Watson–style turnaround, nor access to a Bulgarian health/punishment camp circa 1982, what is the route to better health? The increasingly clear answer from current research is that they should make every effort to become more active, whether in day-to-day life or through exercise, then try to eat a healthy diet and, to an extent, let the weight issues take care of themselves.

Robert Ross says people should be urged to be active because of the overall impact it will have on their health, and be aware that any reductions in weight will most likely be both slow and require significant physical investment. 'If you're doing sixty minutes, five days a week, well, that's pretty good,' he says. 'And if you're not eating more, will you lose weight? Absolutely. But many overweight and obese adults say, "Yes, I'll lose weight, but I'll lose weight slowly. And I wish to lose weight quickly."

'I understand that sentiment, and if someone wishes to lose weight quickly, 5 per cent to 10 per cent of body weight over the next two to three months, they're likely going to need to reduce caloric intake along with physical activity to achieve rapid weight loss. That said, how many more decades of information do we need from across the globe, that large weight losses obtained rapidly are rarely sustained? There's just so much evidence from very well-performed randomised control trials that show substantial weight loss after six and maybe even twelve months, and then there's a gradual recidivism, an erosion of benefit, such that after a couple of years they're right back where they started.'

Part of this, Ross says, is the body's biological response to sustained energy deficits: 'But far more important for the average adult is the recognition that reducing caloric intake substantially, trying to combine that with forty-five or sixty minutes of physical activity most days of the week, is very, very hard to sustain in today's environment, and most adults can't do it.'

People should be reminded that better cardiorespiratory fitness 'is associated with a substantial reduction in morbidity, disease and mortality risk, regardless of the bathroom scale', Ross says. 'That does not, at the same time, suggest that if you lose weight that's a bad idea. There's no question that physical activity is an absolutely essential component of the behavioural mix that adults have to do to sustain any meaningful weight loss – and I think the operative word there is sustained. If you lose some weight or reduce your waist circumference as you're doing that, good for you, but if you don't, still good for you.'

This message is now also starting to come from public health professionals, who are on the front line of grappling with the intertwined crises of inactivity and weight. Dr Justin Varney, whom we heard from earlier, was in charge of adult wellbeing at Public Health England, and now runs public health policy in the city of Birmingham.

'One of the things we have suffered from is perhaps the con-flation of obesity and inactivity,' he says. 'There are lots of other reasons why I'd want you to be physically active, and frankly obesity is not one of them. Physical activity helps you maintain a healthy weight, and it can be an important part of helping you to lose weight. But if you don't fix your diet, you're not going to lose weight. It doesn't work like that. Although I don't like it, the phrase, "You can't outrun a Mars Bar" isn't far off the truth.'[42]

Fat and fit

All this leads us, at last, into the most contentious corner of the activity/weight world, the idea given the catchy, if not entirely satisfactory, title of 'fat and fit', or, if you are being slightly more polite, 'heavy and healthy'. It is an imperfect term in that, as we have seen already, improved physical fitness is worthwhile even if you are overweight, particularly below levels of obesity. The contro-versy comes if you take the idea a step further: is being overweight and active a better health outcome than lean but immobile? One person who is convinced this is the case is Steven Blair, the veteran

South Carolina University academic we encountered earlier in the book, who is among the handful of most eminent and influential researchers into inactivity over the decades.

Blair has carried out numerous studies which compared mortality rates between physical fitness and weight. Perhaps his most famous paper, published in 1999, assessed nearly 22,000 men of various ages with a treadmill test, and measured their body fat percentage. When the data was analysed from more than 400 deaths over an eight-year follow-up period, Blair and his team found that while lean, unfit men had twice the risk of death as fit men of the same body composition, they were also more at risk than men who were fit and obese.[43]

A later study co-authored by Blair assessed the same relationship, but measured not only body fat percentage but also BMI and waist size. This found the latter two measures more significant in bringing a likelihood of early death than fat percentage, but also that fitness (again measured on a treadmill) was even more significant. When the 2,600 participants, all of whom were aged sixty-plus, were split into five bands of descending fitness levels, those in the bottom 20 per cent had four times the risk of death over the twelve-year study period than those in the top quintile. It also found that in the fittest group, even people who were obese, with a BMI of between 30 and 35, had a lower risk of death than those who were normal weight but inactive.[44]

Blair is dismissive of his relatively numerous critics, arguing that many studies which come to other conclusions tend to ask participants to assess their own fitness, or base it on self-reported activity levels. 'You can't lie to the treadmill,' he tells me cheerily over the phone. 'People think I'm absolutely crazy, and we still keep finding the same results, and people attack me and criticise. In the work we have done, obese individuals who are moderately fit and followed over many years are about half as likely to die as normal-weight people who are unfit. I'm not saying we should ignore obesity, and we need to have good strategies for preventing it, and treating it, and all of that. But frankly, it is not nearly as big a public health problem as is inactivity, which leads to low fitness.'

Blair, who is now eighty, admits he has something of a personal stake in the argument: 'To be honest with you, I'm a short, bald, kind of fat guy. I'm also very fit. I get 5 million steps a year. But I've been physically active my whole life. I set that 5 million steps goal and started it on my seventieth birthday. And I've made it every year since then. But it hasn't made me skinny.'[45]

There have been many academic ripostes to Blair's work. One of the best known was a 2004 paper by Harvard academics which used data from a vast and long-term study co-run by the university into US nurses to track the health outcomes of nearly 120,000 women over an average of twenty-four years. This supported the health risks of both excess weight and inactivity, but found that the death risk for obese and active women was about 30 per cent greater than that for those who had a BMI below 25 but moved little.[46]

This is an argument which has run for more than twenty years already, and you could spend a long time poring over the various research papers. And when it comes to everyday life, rather than academic bragging rights, there is an extent to which it is, ultimately, a bit irrelevant. To quote the very straightforward conclusion to the Harvard nurses' study: 'Both increased adiposity [excess weight] and reduced physical activity are strong and independent predictors of death.' Not even Steven Blair would disagree with that, and you would find similar agreement from Robert Ross and Tom Watson, or indeed from more or less anyone who has looked into the intersection between these two gradual, normalised pandemics.

It is beyond doubt that excess weight brings diminished odds for your future health, all the more so when excess weight moves into clinically defined obesity, whether measured by BMI or waist circumference. This has seemingly been shown, recently and tragically, with coronavirus. So, this chapter is not intended to be a clarion call for people to completely ignore excess weight as a potential risk. But the hope is that I can persuade at least some people to view weight in a different light: both as a consequence of the lived environment, and also as something which does not have to be a barrier to fitness.

My own investment in all this is a bit more personal than it was when I began the research. I spent my entire youth very slim, and I was notorious for being able to consume portions of food which bore no apparent relationship to my size. Inevitably, as I have advanced into middle age, what used to definitely be leanness has now become what I like to think of as an average build.

Average is nonetheless a broad term. As we saw in the last chapter, I'm still officially pretty active, if less so than a few years ago. I also work in the Houses of Parliament, a world of odd hours, frequent drinks events and subsidised canteens. It might not officially count as an obesogenic environment, but new MPs are warned by old-timers to beware of too quickly acquiring what is known as the 'Westminster kilo'. I was not exempt. At a recent routine asthma check-up at my doctors' surgery, the nurse looking at my records pointed out that I was in fact two kilos heavier than when last seen, a few years previously.

I was still unbothered when, during the fitness test at Roehampton University described in the last chapter, I was placed in a machine to measure my body fat percentage. This was a high-tech device called a BodPod, a metal canister looking a bit like a 1950s rendition of an alien spaceship. You sit still inside, and the air displaced by your body is measured, which permits a calculation of how much body mass is lean and how much is fat. The results came a few days later. Below the figure for my VO2 max came the reading for body fat. When I saw it, my disappointment at the reduced VO2 max reading was temporarily forgotten: it said I had 30 per cent body fat. For middle-aged men, a few points above 10 per cent is good, and anything up to 20 per cent is acceptable. But 30 per cent put me in the category of not just overweight, but very much obese.

I was simultaneously shocked and a bit frightened, but also baffled. The shock came first: so, I thought, despite all that cycling, my insides are distinctly un-lean. I pored over web pages about reducing body fat, and started to plot a post-book regime of running, weights and a Tom Watson–like no-carb diet.

But most of all I was puzzled. Even with the extra two kilos, my BMI is 22.5, well within the healthy range. My physique looks reasonably lean, clothed or in the bathroom mirror. And for more or less as long as I can remember, I've bought trousers with the same waist size, 31 inches (just under 79cm) – Robert Ross's stated gauge for all being well. What was going on?

Motivated in part by this confusion, but also perhaps by the much more personal wish for a different answer about my supposed interior obesity, I read academic studies about the accuracy of BodPod measurements. These mainly suggested it is accurate, even if a few papers noted occasional anomalous readings.

I needed a second opinion. With the coronavirus lockdown now in place, the only way was via the old-fashioned but still much-used skinfold technique. This uses sprung callipers to measure the thickness of an area of pinched-out skin from a few select places around the body, with the combined total of millimetres converted via online charts into a body fat percentage.

I duly bought some callipers and followed the instructions of various websites as best I could. A very different answer came back: a total of 15 per cent body fat. Not completely lean, no, but perfectly safe.

I was even more bewildered. As a last resort, I emailed Robert Ross and explained my predicament. What should I believe, I asked him? Which method was more accurate? It might seem like overkill – not to mention a bit cheeky – to ask one of the world's leading research experts on excess weight and activity to adjudicate on your own personal obesity issues, but he had seemed very nice on the phone.

Ross very kindly replied, pointing out that it is a complex area, which depends on multiple factors. The BodPod uses a bespoke algorithm within its software to convert the measurement from the air displacement into a reading, he said: 'The bottom line is that *all* field methods of body composition measurement must by design convert some property to whole body fat and/or lean mass scores.' He sent me a link to a study paper by a colleague, nine densely printed pages explaining the many different ways body composition can be determined, packed with charts, tables and formulae.[47] To somewhat oversimplify the study's message, it says: when it comes to body fat, what answer you receive depends in part on what question you ask.

I started to get the idea. So, I wrote in another email to Ross, perhaps I should just assume that my consistent, and healthy, waist size indicated all was probably okay, and I could perhaps just worry a bit less? His very concise reply came two minutes later: 'Amen, Peter.'

As a final lesson for this chapter, my brief if still unresolved brush with clinical obesity could hardly be more fitting. Yes, it is easy to become complacent about weight, and if your activity level does drop even a bit, as mine had, you can't rely on your appetite to reduce in turn. But ultimately, if you remain active, it can be easy to get lost in a tangle of different, competing measurements.

If there is one message that needs to be better and more widely conveyed, it is to dispel the idea that there is not much point trying to become active if you are overweight. Relatively few people can manage the feats of Tom Watson. Many more could benefit from embracing the ethos of Robert Ross: become active, forget about the scales for a bit, and just see what happens.

Next steps

Weight and obesity is such a hugely complex and involved subject, but if there's one message that resonated with me in writing this chapter, it was that of Jean Mayer: if it comes to a choice between permanently reducing your food intake and being more active, the latter is often easier, not to mention more fun.

7

Your Everyday Life is Dangerous

If, by any chance, you ever make a speech to a conference populated mainly by public health experts, and at the end they all leap to their feet to applaud, by all means feel satisfied. But don't get too smug. This could be the phenomenon known as 'active applause'. This dictates that every speaker receives a standing ovation, not because they are necessarily brilliant, simply as a reminder to the audience to stand up and move around between the presentations. These are the people who have studied the consequences of prolonged sitting more closely than anyone else. Should we pay attention to the fact that they start to get a bit nervy if forced to sit down for more than twenty minutes or so at a time? I think we probably should.

Like most people, I have been at least generally aware for a while that too much sitting down isn't the best idea for your health. Sitting, the newspaper feature story headlines proclaim, is the new smoking. As someone who has for more than two decades been in a job, journalism, much of which is done using a chair, I also knew this idea had some personal relevance to me. I was particularly struck by the notion of active applause, explained to me by an academic a few years ago. I must sit down less, I mentally told myself at the time, while not really making any plans as to how this might happen.

Sitting is, along with Chapter 5's focus on walking, cycling and stair climbing, probably the way in which the modern world has most carefully conspired against our biological inheritance as active creatures. But, like those, it is also the area where it is often possible to make the most life-enhancing changes. Make no mistake, for all that the 'new smoking' headlines overstate the case – unlike tobacco, chairs and sofas don't kill 1 per cent or so of their users every year[1] – there is no doubt that prolonged, particularly uninterrupted sitting, if maintained over decades, does significantly worsen your health odds. While it often coincides with more general inactivity, and many of the health perils cross over between the two, sitting down is a distinct issue and one often not properly understood. It is also more complex than just plonking one's bum on a seat. Not all types of sitting are the same, and some are definitely worse than others.

To begin with the terminological basics, sedentary behaviour, as distinct from general physical inactivity, describes not just a lack of motion or exertion, but a body that is seated or prone, although not asleep. In clinical terms it is thus possible for someone to be excessively sedentary but not classified as inactive. For example, they might go for a reasonably long run every morning, and then even cycle to work, but sit at a desk for ten hours. Less common but still achievable is to not be deemed sedentary but nonetheless still be classified as inactive, for example a person who stands behind a till in a shop for their job, but moves very little over the course of their day.

As well as sitting (or lying), being sedentary also means not moving around too much while you do it. The standard academic definition is 'any waking behaviour characterised by an energy expenditure of less than 1.5 METs while in a sitting, reclining or lying posture'.[2] Although 1.5 METs is 50 per cent more energy than that needed for someone's body to just tick over, it is small enough to cover most seated tasks. One study which tested this out found that even typing or playing video games kept people, on average, below the 1.5 MET level, with the only exception being a Nintendo Wii–type game in which the controller was waved around to play. Standing up, in contrast, immediately nudged people into the territory of 1.6 METs.[3]

Sustained sitting down might seem entirely natural to the vast majority of modern people, but it's worth remembering that the common use of chairs, let alone habitual sedentariness, is a fairly modern development. In a fascinating book which tracks the way the human body has altered with different ways of living over the millennia, *Primate Change*, the UK academic Vybarr Cregan-Reid makes the point that while chairs have existed for thousands of years, for many centuries they were so rare as to be commonly associated with power or authority – hence the use of 'chair' as the highest title in a university.[4]

When, in the more distant past, people wanted to rest for a period, a common method was to squat on their haunches. This is something occasionally seen today, but generally only in parts of East and Southeast Asia. The majority of chair-habituated adults tend to find squatting for any period fairly uncomfortable. From the bitter professional experience of trying to perch just above a wet pavement but out of the view of TV cameras to take notes while a politician gives a statement, I know I can generally last only a few minutes without having to shift. Cregan-Reid argues that years of daily sitting has so shortened most people's hip flexors, the bands of muscle around the joint, that their pelvis is permanently tilted forwards, even when standing – an adaptation he believes contributes to the epidemic of back pain in many nations.[5]

The rise of the chair as the default support for the human body has happened on two fronts. In the home, comfortable upholstering using fabric emerged in the early eighteenth century, particularly in the French royal court, even though a combination of cost and generally damp houses limited its initial spread. Far more influential was the Industrial Revolution and the dawn of the seated, urbanised workforce. English census figures show the pace of change. Between 1851 and 1871 the number of commercial clerks shot up from just under 44,000 to more than 91,000. Office work still remained a minority occupation in an era with more than 110,000 blacksmiths and a million-plus servants. But the trajectory was obvious. In 1851, England had almost 1.5 million farm labourers and shepherds. Twenty years later that figure had fallen to 980,000.[6]

And now? In many countries, sitting down has become the norm for large parts of the day, both at work and during leisure. Precise figures vary, not least because much of the data is self-assessed, but various surveys have claimed common figures for the UK of up to nine hours of sitting time a day,[7] a figure matched by estimates in places like Australia.[8] The most recent NHS figures are slightly less dramatic, saying that around a third of adults sit for six hours a day or more on weekdays, with a slightly higher figure at weekends. An international study, which took data from twenty countries, found an average daily sitting time of five hours. This varied between countries, with Portugal, Brazil and Colombia reporting averages below this, while Norway, Japan, Saudi Arabia, Taiwan and Hong Kong saw greater than six hours.[9]

What does seem common is that when the researchers are able to actually measure how long people are immobile, rather than just asking them, the hours involved start to rise. US researchers enlisted more than 8,000 middle-aged and older people to wear a movement-monitoring device during the day for up to a week. It found that sedentary behaviour took up more than 75 per cent of people's entire days on average, totalling more than eleven hours. In contrast, those tested were lightly active, for example standing up or walking around, for about three hours a day, and managed an average of around eighteen minutes of moderate or vigorous exertion. The authors did note that this particular set of figures could be higher than the US average because around half the data was collected in the chillingly named Stroke Belt, a collection of southeastern states including Alabama, Kentucky, Tennessee and North and South Carolina which suffer particularly high rates of both strokes and early death, something closely connected to poverty levels as well as inactive, sedentary living.[10]

For all that the idea of active applause made me think about sitting down, it's fair to say it still didn't make much of an immediate dent in my behaviour. Soon after learning about it, I moved into the specialism of political journalism. This was in the aftermath of the UK's Brexit referendum, a period involving two general elections, two changes of prime minister and near-constant drama and chaos. It certainly felt to me like I was spending a long time sitting in my office chair, typing up the latest developments. But how long?

So, again, I decided to become my own research subject. To make sure the data was robust, it couldn't just be about me making estimates. So I went in search of some technology. There are plenty of mass-market activity trackers that will try to assess how many minutes a day you have spent sitting down, but they tend to have drawbacks. Phone apps are, as we saw with the data in earlier chapters on step counts, reliant on someone carrying the device. But more than that, in measuring activity, both smartphones and wrist-based trackers like Fitbits, as well as the Garmin smartwatch I borrowed to measure my heart rate, use in-built accelerometers, sensors which measure acceleration forces, and thus movement. To work out whether someone is sitting, standing, walking or running, this raw data must be interpreted, and to an extent it depends where on the body the device is located. This makes phones, at best, approximate arbiters of step counts, let alone sitting time. Even wrist-based movement sensors have their limitations in this regard. In a break writing an earlier part of this chapter, I remained sitting down but spent a minute or so swinging my left arm back and forth, promptly registering another hundred-plus steps for the on-screen daily tally. I needed something accurate enough to be used in laboratory tests.

Internet searching led me to the website of a small Danish company called Sens, which manufactures tiny devices that look a bit like the plastic security tags you see on clothes in shops, but much smaller, weighing just seven grams.[11] Using a bespoke plaster they are attached to the outside of the thigh, just above the knee, where the measurements for acceleration and angle can be much more easily translated into accurate assessments of walking, standing, sitting and other behaviours. They are waterproof and can be left on for days, even weeks at a time. Intrigued, I sent a speculative email to the address listed on the website, explaining that rather than being a university researcher hoping to buy a few hundred sensors (their usual customer), I was an author who wanted just one sensor, for me. Oh yes, and I didn't really know what I was doing. I was doubtful how interested they would be.

A few days later, however, the company's joint founder, Kasper Lykkegaard, emailed back to say they would happily sell me a single device, with full technical support, for a bargain price. He even arranged a video call so he could talk me through how to attach the sensor and access the data. It stores up to two weeks' information at a time, which can be downloaded to the company's website, via the intermediary of a smartphone app. If you are a professional you can see this in raw accelerometer form, or a graph showing the angle the device is pointed at over time.

Luckily for me the website also turns all this information into an easily digestible 24-hour rolling bar chart. Each hour is split into fifteen-minute chunks which then rise upwards, divided in turn into various bands of colour, depending on what the wearer has been doing. Standing is marked in blue, walking is orange, and what is termed intermittent walking – what you might call pottering around – comes as a sort of yellow. The most satisfying colours are a bright green for running, and a darker green to indicate cycling. And then there is sitting or lying, represented as a blank, featureless grey.

Luckily, I obtained the sensor some weeks before the coronavirus emergency began in the UK, and so I was able to wear it for a few weeks during my normal pattern of working. One of the rules of science is that when something is observed it necessarily changes, so I decided to, essentially, attach the device to my leg and try to forget about it. It was so tiny that this was just what happened. Of course, I can't rule out some half-conscious awareness that might have made me more likely to, say, break up a prolonged period in my chair, but in general this felt like the natural, workplace me.

When I did examine the results, even though I knew I had a job where I could and should stand up more, there was still a significantly larger mass of sedentary grey on the charts than expected. One immediate contrast was the difference between workdays and weekends. The latter showed occasional sustained periods of sitting, mainly at mealtimes, and again later in the evenings. But for the most part, it was continually broken up by flashes of colour to indicate walking and standing, even brief bursts of vivid green for running, mainly playing football in the local park with my son.

In contrast, the charts for workdays were much more drab, even given the morning-and-evening periods of cycling green for my commute. This was a fairly relentlessly busy news period, amid the combined news pressures of the latest Brexit fallout and the build-up to coronavirus. But it seemed no more busy than the rest of the near-four years I have spent reporting from Westminster, and so the sensor data was probably typical. As such, it was pretty depressing.

Yes, there were fairly regular periods of walking, every day. Weeks earlier, Downing Street officials had changed the location of the twice-daily briefing with the prime minister's spokesman, moving it from inside parliament to an office in 11 Downing Street, an extra ten-minute walk away. We had cursed the inconvenience at the time, but looking back at my activity record, it did at least generate a reasonably long orange bar for walking. But the later the chart went into any workday, the longer and more damning became the grey gaps between bursts of movement. Even in the internet era, newspaper time pressures tend to tilt towards a late afternoon deadline to deliver copy for the next day's physical paper, and after lunch it was common to see two-hour periods in which I had clearly been out of my office chair not once, or very briefly, just sitting there, typing. Overall, the whole period from about 2pm to 6:30pm or so tended to be a long line of grey.

Seeing my days presented as such an eloquent, easy-to-understand activity chronicle was simultaneously fascinating and alarming, and sometimes in ways that highlighted other sedentary aspects of modern life, those outside the office. For example, the day I travelled to Copenhagen to interview Jan Gehl, whom we heard from in Chapter 5, I spent much of it walking and cycling around the city, splashing the chart in satisfying orange and green. But it also showed a long, unbroken grey period when I was sitting down on the flight from London.

The Sens software allows you to download the full data as a chart for each day, with a combined total for each type of movement, and a step count. It's fair to say the picture, particularly for workdays, was mixed. I would rack up half an hour or so of cycling – my actual commute takes more like thirty-five minutes there and back, but waiting at traffic lights and junctions would be measured as standing – and my step count would somehow generally top 10,000. On my day tramping around Copenhagen I amassed a barely plausible 20,000 steps. But then there was the sitting. Here, the data showed two problems. Firstly, there were prolonged immobile periods, not broken up by standing or walking, a pattern which, as we'll see later, is believed to be particularly hazardous.

Also, there was the sheer amount of sitting down. The sensor does not distinguish between sitting and sleeping, but captures every single sedentary moment, from a brief sit-down to an office chair marathon. And, for me, it really added up. Even after discounting the time spent in bed, I would regularly clock up nine hours or more of immobile time every workday. Even on what looked like busy, active weekend days it could easily reach five or six hours.

I was officially sedentary. Yes, I was also active, at least by government guidelines – as we saw in Chapter 5, my commute into work alone takes me well above the minimum thresholds. But in health terms, did the latter cancel out the former? I needed to find out.

Throw away your television

The physiological reasons why prolonged sitting is bad for you are very similar in many ways to the risk factors for inactivity in general, but to an extent they are more condensed. We saw earlier how regular movement helps your body transport and process different types of fat, including high-density lipoprotein cholesterol (HDL) – the 'good' cholesterol – and variants linked with poorer health outcomes, mainly low-density lipoprotein cholesterol (LDL) and triglycerides.

The significance of prolonged sitting is that it puts some of our biggest muscles, notably in the legs and the back, into a cellular process known as downregulation, during which they produce less of certain proteins. These muscles are among the sort known as 'red muscles', so called because they are rich in capillaries, and are resistant to fatigue. They contain disproportionately high levels of lipoprotein lipase, which has a major role in breaking down triglycerides.

Low-intensity activity, such as standing up or walking around, is a biological signal for this work to take place. If someone stays sitting down, this fat processing doesn't happen properly, bringing a greater risk of cardiovascular disease, as well as excess weight. A body which does not properly break down triglycerides also has a higher chance of being unable to correctly process glucose, which is the path leading towards type 2 diabetes.

At the most basic biological level these risks have been demonstrated using unpleasant-sounding laboratory experiments in which rats had their rear legs suspended above the floor for sustained periods over eleven days. The scientists found that these underused leg muscles ended up with significantly lower levels of lipoprotein lipase than those of rats not subjected to the regime.[12]

While researchers are not permitted to treat human volunteers in quite the same way, reading some academic papers it can sometimes be hard to notice much of a difference. Numerous studies have used what is usually known as 'bed rest' – lying down for as much of the day as possible beyond basic bodily functions – to show the numerous ways that complete sedentariness affects the body. One 1968 experiment, which would presumably struggle to pass ethical guidelines now, saw five young American male volunteers spend a marathon twenty continuous days in bed. At the end of this, their fitness was almost a third lower than at the start, and even their hearts had shrunk by 11 per cent. Luckily, the researchers then put them all through an eight-week fitness programme, which undid the damage.[13]

In population-wide terms, the consequences of prolonged sitting are also well proven, and the risks are many. A massive study published in 2018 tracked more than 127,000 US men and women over an average of twenty-one years, assessing them on the basis of non-work sitting. Those who averaged six hours or more sitting per day had significantly worse health prospects than those whose average was less than three hours. For more habitual sitters, the study concluded, the risks were higher in terms of dying for any reasons, and for acquiring cardiovascular disease and strokes, cancer, diabetes, kidney disease, chronic obstructive pulmonary disease (COPD), liver disease, digestive problems, Parkinson's, Alzheimer's, musculoskeletal disorders, nervous disorders and suicide.[14]

This is quite a list, even if it is perhaps fair to argue that, even with other variables factored out, prolonged sitting can still be a decent proxy for more general inactivity. One particular academic focus over the years has been on the perils of watching television, and the conclusions are more or less always the same – the more you watch, the worse your chances.

A UK study with a cohort of just over 13,000 people in Norfolk found that after the standard adjustments for other factors, each one-hour increase in average daily viewing time increased people's overall chances of death during the study by 5 per cent, and the risk of cardiovascular disease by 8 per cent.[15] Other research has indicated that the risks can then escalate. A US paper which tracked more than 220,000 fifty-plus adults for an average of fourteen years found that when compared to those who watched less than an hour a day, people who averaged three and a half hours – which, the researchers noted, is the norm for 80 per cent of Americans, taking up half their entire leisure time – had a 15 per cent higher chance of death for any reason over the course of the research. For the group who racked up an admittedly formidable seven hours or more a day, the additional mortality risk went up to 47 per cent. This covered eight separate increased health risks: cancer, cardiovascular disease, COPD, diabetes, flu or pneumonia, Parkinson's, liver disease and suicide. 'There was no cause of death where TV viewing was protective,' the authors added, perhaps unnecessarily.[16]

According to Dr Katrien Wijndaele, an epidemiologist and research scientist at Cambridge University, who led the Norfolk study, television viewing tends to show a generally worse series of health outcomes even compared to other sedentary behaviours, for example office work. There are, she says, several theories as to why this might be the case, all of which could be at least partly true. One, she explains, could be because, as mentioned earlier, watching a lot of TV 'is just one of those behaviours that tends to be higher in people who also show many more other unhealthy behaviours', and that studies are unable to properly account for all these other activities. Connected to that is research showing that when people watch TV they are more exposed to advertisements for unhealthy foods and snacks, which could affect their diet and thus further embed their existing non-TV health risks.

On a biological level, the bulk of TV viewing tends to happen in the evening, generally after people have eaten their biggest and most sugar- and fat-laden meal of the day. As we have seen before, being inactive in this so-called postprandial state can worsen the way our bodies process fats and sugars, with long-term results for our cardiovascular systems and chances of moving towards pre-diabetes.

There is a final theory: all sedentary time is more or less equally bad, but TV watching comes across worse in the studies because it's the only one that people report correctly. 'We find that TV viewing tends to be recalled better by people, because it's done in a very habitual way,' Wijndaele says. 'People basically remember programmes they watch, and so they can fairly accurately report on levels of TV viewing, more accurately compared to other types of sitting. Sitting is something we do throughout the day. We can't remember when we go and sit down, when we get up again. So if you ask people about a total estimate of their sitting time, or even of other, more specific types of sitting, it's a lot harder to recall those. So if you then have to come up with a total estimate of sitting time, they tend to be less valid and reliable than estimates of TV viewing time. So that is one factor that could explain why we find those stronger associations for TV viewing.'[17]

Whether or not television is being unfairly maligned, it is accepted more generally that not all sitting behaviours are the same, and that some versions could be more harmful than others. In the most basic sense, that's perhaps obvious. For example, it is little surprise that a movement-based computer game like a Nintendo Wii takes people above 1.5 METs when other computer games do not. Waving your arms about needs more exertion than just pushing buttons with your thumbs, whether or not you are sitting on a sofa at the time.

There are workplace equivalents. In *Primate Change*, Vybarr Cregan-Reid cites studies in Sardinia which showed that women living there who were tailors or seamstresses generally enjoyed good health despite their sedentary work. The reason appeared to be that they used pedal-operated manual sewing machines, with the leg action providing the women with sufficient levels of exertion, as well as, the researchers found, notably muscular calves.[18]

More widely, there are also suggestions that sitting in leisure time can be worse for your health than doing it at work. Danish research from 2016 found people who habitually used a chair in their job but sat less at home were more likely to have better fitness and smaller waist sizes than those whose sitting was mainly done out of the office.[19] A series of studies by Swedish academics have made an actual distinction between 'passive' sedentary behaviour, for example watching television, or 'active' sitting, such as if you read or sit at a computer.[20]

There is perhaps a danger here of stigmatising one type of sitting, not least as numerous studies have shown that – as you might expect – lengthy sitting time in the workplace is more associated with middle-class jobs. In contrast, poorer people tend to watch more television.

Others, however, argue that the differences between types of sitting go well beyond this. James Levine, a British researcher who has spent most of his career in America, is one of the most regular public voices warning about the perils of prolonged sitting. He has written a book, *Get Up!*,[21] an enjoyable half scientific autobiography, half diatribe against the modern curse that he calls 'chairdom'. Levine clearly enjoys his role as something of an academic maverick, at one point in the book recounting how a failed experiment had started a fire, adding, nonchalantly: 'Anyway, it wasn't the first lab I had blown up.'[22]

Levine's research breakthrough, first outlined in a paper just over twenty years ago, was something he calls 'non-exercise activity thermogenesis', or NEAT. This argues that even when immobile, different people expend significantly varying amounts of energy through activities they might not even realise they are doing, such as foot tapping, arm and leg swinging, and other fidgeting, or brushing back their hair, perhaps picking up a magazine to flick through it. In keeping with his individualistic approach, Levine tracked people's movements using what he styled as 'magic underpants', high-tech devices fitted with sensors to detect what people were doing.

Levine's initial paper calculated that even while sitting, someone who is fidgeting can expend over 50 per cent more energy than a person who is motionless in a chair. The amounts are fairly small – about 2.5 calories per minute – but they add up if extended over some hours.[23] In a follow-up experiment a year later, Levine enlisted sixteen non-obese volunteers, himself among them, to eat an extra 1,000 calories above what was calculated as each person's weight-maintenance food intake for a full eight weeks. While, as you might expect, everyone gained weight, the amounts involved varied from about a third of a kilo to over 4kg. The participants' NEAT expenditure was measured again, thanks to the magic underwear, and was also found to vary hugely in response to the overfeeding, with high NEAT levels corresponding with low weight gains. Sadly for Levine, among the discoveries he made was that he was not among those people who can fidget their way to eating what they like.[24] NEAT is, of course, not just about movement while sitting. The overfeeding trial showed that participants who gained the most weight sat on average for over two hours a day more than those who did not. But it demonstrates how not all sitting is equal in health terms.

To a layperson this can feel similar to the folk wisdom that slim people have a 'higher metabolic rate' than those who gain weight. But studies have shown this idea seems to be a myth. Basal metabolic rate, the amount of energy someone's body consumes when immobile, varies between people for a variety of reasons, including gender and the proportion of muscle mass, but actually tends to be higher in overweight and obese people.[25] Remaining slim is not some in-built biological given – it is all about different amounts of movement, even movements people don't always notice in everyday life, like regularly standing up, or fidgeting.

Speaking from Paris, where he is now based, Levine told me that his ideas were first met with incredulity from the research community. Before the initial paper was published, Levine says, he presented its findings to a conference, at the end of which a very senior academic – whom he does not name – stood up and said: 'This is a total load of rubbish!'

As it turned out, Levine's paper was picked up by the prestigious US journal *Science,* and the sceptical academic ended up collaborating on a future piece of work. Levine says the consensus on the idea is now clear: 'I think now, much more the greater question is the one of, how do we really implement this society-wide?'

Given the impracticality of persuading people to spend hours a day fidgeting, Levine's solution is for activity to be built into other areas of life, including active travel. He argues that a combination of the inactivity crisis and the climate emergency should be used as an opportunity to completely reshape cities in favour of walking and cycling, and he would like to see his adopted home, Paris, make itself entirely car-free: 'When big things happen in societies, it's rarely one thing that precipitates big change, it's normally the collision of several things.'[26]

Levine was being more prescient than he could have realised. We spoke just before the coronavirus emergency descended. At time of writing, to cope with the socially distanced transport aftermath, Paris's mayor, Anne Hidalgo, has removed cars from a series of city centre roads and announced plans for hundreds of miles of extra cycle lanes. Levine's dream could be about to happen.

Don't just sit there

One of the biggest risks from excessive sitting down is known to be a greater propensity to diabetes, as well as the associated risk of increased waist size. Yet again, television viewing appears as a particularly significant factor, with one joint British–Australian project concluding that it contributed to twice the diabetes risk of sedentary time at work.[27] One very long-term Swedish study found a clear link between the extent of television viewing among test subjects when they were sixteen and biological indicators showing their susceptibility to diabetes when they were forty-three.[28]

Professor David Dunstan, who heads the physical activity laboratory at the Baker Heart and Diabetes Institute in Melbourne, is one of the world's leading experts on the dangers of too much sitting time, and has led several studies about the connection to diabetes. There is, he says, a 'sound biological rationale' for the link: 'The absence of muscle contraction that occurs through long hours of sitting is not favourable for the whole glucose transport process. So, what we do know is that just muscle action itself can greatly help in terms of clearing glucose from the bloodstream. It's pretty well documented in the epidemiological literature that regular physical activity in addition to other life-style factors like diet is an important modifier of risk for type 2 diabetes development.'[29]

Despite my many hours in the office chair I don't, as far as I know, have any clinical signs linking me with diabetes. But both the amount of time I sit, and my unusually high, if bit-terly contested, body fat reading would seemingly increase my risks of heading down that path. The two are also connected, with numerous studies linking sedentary lives with all sorts of obesity-related gauges, whether BMI, waist circumference or body fat percentage.

So what can I do about it? There is something fairly imme-diate, it seems – make sure that even if I do sit down a lot, that time is at least interrupted fairly regularly. This is yet another way, as also highlighted in James Levine's studies, in which not all sitting is the same. In terms of inactivity science, this is still relatively new, but the evidence is now very strong that one of the best ways to ameliorate the biological problems that come from prolonged sitting is to make sure that every now and then you jerk your bodily system into action, whether just by stand-ing up, or ideally going for a wander, even just to get a cup of tea or to talk to a colleague.

One Australian study – a disproportionate amount of aca-demic work on the health risks of sitting time seems to take place in Australia and the UK – fitted movement sensors to a group of middle-aged volunteers to assess how often they took a break from sitting, judged in this case as at least a minute of movement. Those who sat for the same overall time, but got up less often, were found to have more indicators of a propensity to diabetes, as well as bigger waists. In fact, when the group was split into quarters according to how often they broke their sit-ting, those in the 25 per cent who got up the least regularly had, on average, a 6cm bigger waist than those who did it the most.[30] The risks seem to go further. One later US project tracking nearly 8,000 middle-aged US people found that both prolonged sitting time and long bouts of continuous sitting were linked to the risk of early death. Those who did the two faced the greatest dangers.[31] One thing must be added: while simply standing up does use those vital leg and back muscles, it does not necessarily count as something sufficiently vigorous to break up sitting. A UK study which measured insulin and glucose levels in people who sat for long periods after a meal found that while these were improved in people who walked around for a few minutes every half an hour, there was no discernible effect on those who simply stood up.[32]

Professor Genevieve Healy is a researcher at the School of Public Health in Australia's Queensland University, and led some of the pioneering studies showing the benefits of breaking up prolonged sitting. She says the initial findings confirmed what she had suspected as an 'observational epidemiologist'. She tells me: 'I used to be quite a sitter and happily sit and not fidget and just happily sit all day. And then my boss couldn't sit still. But he had to sit in a lot of meetings. So I was like, "I wonder if there's any difference between him and me in terms of out-comes? I wonder if we can capture that sort of thing in people that we actually put good monitors on and measured all their biomarkers." And that's when the results came back. There's a bit of common sense as well, because if you get to the movies, or you get stuck in a car or plane for a long time, you can feel that difference between when you do that, versus when you're getting up regularly. So I call it filling in the evidence for some common sense science.'[33]

There is an extent to which Healy's boss is an example of James Levine's high-NEAT fidgeters, people who in this case are so restless they don't just tap a foot but intermittently get up and march around. Healy says she has now changed her own habits: 'Probably the most I can sit is twenty minutes before I start to get quite fidgety, so I have a sit–stand desk at work, and that's made a massive difference because I can just work in whatever posture I like. But in our workplace we've been doing this for over a decade – we've trained our building to be very aware of all the benefits of regular changes in posture, so nobody bats an eyelid if you get up, and most people get up and down during meetings, so it's seen as natural. When we have speakers, people get up and down. It's not seen as rude or anything.'

Healy is at the forefront of examining ways workplaces can reduce sitting time. She led a project at one office involving sit–stand workstations, which can be placed either at traditional desk height or propelled upwards so people can stand and work. This saw sitting time reduced by an average of three hours per eight-hour workday within three months, even if it did slip to a 45-minute reduction after a year. Reading the study, however, shows the amount of effort needed for such results – it was not just a matter of installing the new desks. The process began with meetings involving managers across the workplace (a federal government agency) and included individual training sessions for everyone given a new desk, plus regular phone consultations to make sure they were being used properly.[34]

Her university is behind an Australia-wide programme called BeUpstanding, which offers web-based support to workplaces wanting to reduce sitting times. This is not as comprehensive as the experiment at the government agency, but the results are still impressive. Since the scheme started in 2017, around 350 workplaces have signed up, with an average reduction in seated time of 9 per cent, or forty minutes a day.

'It's pretty good for predominantly just an education and

culture change programme,' Healy says. 'There had been a lot of media in Australia about too much sitting for quite a long time because we've been doing a lot of the leading research and so a lot of workplaces invested in sit–stand workstations, but then there was no culture change behind that. They put this money in, got the workstations, and then people were like, "What are these for? Why should I use them?" So they just weren't using them, despite this big investment.'

Another option is to reconfigure workspaces to ensure people get up fairly regularly and go for at least a brief walk. As we saw in the last chapter, some of this is about the design of the building, such as Google's system of first-floor workspaces and ground-floor toilets. But it can be much more simple than that, as Healy explains: 'One of our more popular strategies is having a rule of no lunch at the desk. That's a free strategy that people can do. It also helps create a culture where you're meeting, talking together, creating a stronger bond.' This is a common observation – that encouraging people to get up more in an office doesn't just make them healthier, it also improves communication around the office.

One of the key principles of the BeUpstanding project is that staff get to decide what methods work best for them. One of Healy's favourite examples came in a call centre where she helped implement a programme to reduce sitting time. It was, she recalls, 'a very high-stress environment' where abusive calls were relatively regular. 'One of the strategies that their team chose was that if someone got an abusive call, they would stand up and shake it off,' Healy says. 'And what that also meant, obviously, was that other people could see that experience, the abusive call, and check in on them. And so it actually had quite an impact on stress reduction as well as sitting time.'

As you might expect, James Levine has numerous ideas about

how to discourage sitting at work, everything from switching around the location codes for printers, so a department's printer is in a different part of the building, to entirely redesigning offices around open stairwells, providing an impetus for people to walk and chat to colleagues.

But often, he argues, the simplest and cheapest ideas can be the most effective. At the scientific think tank in Paris where he now works, meetings or phone calls can be colour-coded in green on the shared office calendar, meaning they are done on the move. Levine's call with me was one of these, he says, and so he talked while walking up and down the office. Such designations are 'not a reminder but an obligation', he says, and different parts of the organisation compete against each other to see who can have the highest percentage of green meetings. There are even special 'Walking meeting in progress' lanyards to wear, so if you are talking to someone in person others don't interrupt or eavesdrop. 'All of these things we've just talked about cost nothing,' Levine says. 'On the other hand, building an entire building around a stairwell is a feat of engineering.'[35]

For those not working in so forward-thinking an environment, there are of course technological prompts people can use. For example, the heart rate–reading, step-counting exercise watch I borrowed for this book beeps and vibrates on my wrist to warn if I have been sitting down for an hour without a break. Most such devices have similar alerts built in. With mine, I do often find myself responding by jumping from a chair or the sofa to walk around the room. Less expensively, there are a range of apps or programmes which will nudge you to get up at regular intervals via an alert, or a pop-up window on your computer. Some initial studies have indicated that such reminders can help people be more active. But it is by no means certain that this amounts to anything more than an extra tool to help people who have already decided to move around more anyway.

There are experts who worry that too much of the debate about sitting down ends up missing the point. Dr Justin Varney, the wellbeing expert we heard from in the last chapter, who now runs public health for the city of Birmingham, warns that the subject has 'a complete over-focus' on middle-class people in office jobs, who are often not the most sedentary overall.

'The people we need most to be physically active are not sedentary because they're sat in an office,' he says. 'They're sedentary because they're sat at home, they're lonely and they're isolated. They're watching TV or on a computer. Ultimately it's a bit like trying to ban coffee, or put alcohol back in the box. If someone says to me, "Well, you can't binge-watch *Picard*, or whatever you're into at the moment," I'd be very indignant and I'd tell them to sod off. We need to be realistic about what we can change and what we can't. I think this is a distraction. We should be focusing much more on getting everybody active every day, and I don't care how you get moving.'[36]

In population-wide campaigning terms, Varney could well be correct. But if you are someone, like me, who does sit down a lot for work, that doesn't mean you should ignore the issue. During my research, whenever I spoke on the phone to an academic or researcher connected to inactivity science, I would always ask them if they were speaking from a sit–stand desk. They invariably were.

One of my activity-based pledges to myself, when I finish this book – assuming the coronavirus lockdown ever eases enough for me to regularly return to my office in Westminster – is to ask my newspaper to get me a sit–stand desk. That I've not done this so far is partly down to sheer practicality. The Houses of Parliament can be a magical place to work, but some of the conditions, especially in the upper-floor corridor reserved for the media, can be quite basic. Our newspaper is crammed into a fairly poky room, and my worry is that a sit–stand desk will simply not fit into my corner, or would simply bash against one of the ancient bookcases when I tried to raise it. Elsewhere, however, these desks are becoming more common. Ever the individualist, James Levine has gone a stage further and invented the treadmill desk, a standing desk where you walk as you work on a conveyor belt, like that seen on indoor running machines. These are even better for your health outcomes and have a core of enthusiastic users, even if some reports note that it can make drinking coffee slightly perilous.

Another complication is that, at the time of writing, many more people are not just working from home, but look set to be doing so for some months, perhaps even indefinitely as companies realise how much they can save on commercial rents. If the ergonomics of an office can be tricky, creating a movement-friendly work environment at the kitchen table or in your bedroom is even more challenging.

But there was one more question about my sedentary life I wanted to know. If I do ever resume my usual three-and-a-half-mile daily bike commute to and from Westminster, will the physical exertion of the cycling cancel out all health risks of prolonged sitting down?

Research would seem to indicate it should at least mitigate some of it. Probably the most thorough answer so far was published in *The Lancet* in 2016. A Norwegian–Australian–American co-production, this was a meta-study that pulled together data from dozens of papers on the risks of sitting and of inactivity, totalling more than a million people. In good news for me, it found that for people in the highest 25 per cent for physical activity, a category my commute alone would propel me into, the risks of early death were no different between those who sat for less than four hours a day and those who averaged more than eight hours.[37]

But I wanted some outside confirmation. So I sent Professor David Dunstan a series of charts downloaded from my activity tracker showing a fairly typical week in the Westminster office and from a weekend. How worried should I be, I asked him? The reply arrived a few days later, with Dunstan correctly guessing from the charts that I did not have a sit–stand desk. 'Your pattern is fairly typical for an office worker, with the exception that you are highly active,' he said, hearteningly, even adding a cheery, 'Well done!' to the fact the read-outs somehow showed me averaging more than 10,000 steps a day, a total assisted by trips to the twice-daily Downing Street press briefings, and the eccentric layout of the parliamentary estate, which means I can walk for five minutes to fetch a coffee or get some lunch.

There were, however, some caveats. Dunstan noticed that particularly during weekdays there were periods of up to two hours at a time in which I would barely move. 'As a general guide, one should try to take a break from sitting every thirty minutes,' he wrote. 'You mostly achieve this, but there were a couple of periods that this wasn't the case. We call these "danger zones" with our workers and attempt to get them to identify such zones and make adjustments.'[38]

These were resonant words. Yes, my commute, plus the fact that, as the activity tracker shows, I have a tendency to walk more than I perhaps realise, does bring protection. But two hours without a break is a very long time for blood-filled, lipoprotein-rich leg and back muscles to stay essentially dormant, drastically scaling back their vital role in the processing of sugars and fats. Things needed to change.

I don't want to present my working and writing life since then as a revolution, one in which I have eliminated huge parts of my sitting time with a James Levine-like zeal. Banished from the office and without access to a standing desk, let alone a treadmill one, I have had to improvise. Much of the writing of this book has taken place in a borrowed flat fairly close to where I live. It is temporarily uninhabited – hence I could borrow it – and thus unfurnished. I brought with me an old table and chair, where I still spend a reasonable amount of the writing day. But I have tried, wherever possible, to mix things up, perching my laptop on whatever surface is about the correct height, adjusted as needed by a pile of hefty physical activity textbooks. This has included the kitchen worktop and the top of a built-in cupboard by the front door. I'm typing these words with the computer leaned precariously on a windowsill, wobbling slightly if I press a key with too much emphasis. This is still all very conscious, prompted sometimes by the beeping of the smart watch. But with luck, by the time the writing is finished, it could have become a habit.

As I've said before, this book isn't meant to be a guidebook to better health. I'm also aware that there is a chance a reasonable proportion of readers will already be quite physically active. If so, this chapter might be the moment to really start paying attention. You might walk, run, cycle or otherwise Zumba well beyond the 150 recommended minutes a week, but being too sedentary can bring its own risks, and it can be alarmingly easy to overlook. After all, it's just a matter of sitting down.

Next steps:

Given the many knock-on changes from coronavirus, even after lockdown ends it seems likely that many people will work from home more often, which can be a challenge for sitting time. If few offices have sit–stand desks, even fewer homes do. And going to your kitchen to make lunch isn't even as much movement as a walk to a sandwich shop or canteen. So try to find ways to stand up to work at home, if you can. I've now bought a fairly cheap laptop stand with adjustable, folding legs. If I set it to the right height on a table, I can stand to type. I try to alternate – one hour sitting, one hour standing.

8

Youth, Age, and Why Activity Matters Lifelong

It's fair to say that the initiative which has perhaps most improved the physical fortunes of British children over recent years had an unlikely catalyst. It was 2012, and Nigel Buchanan, a retired solicitor, was volunteering at St Ninian's primary school in Stirling, central Scotland. The 79-year-old led after-school chess clubs, taught children the penny whistle and organised outdoor adventure courses in the grounds of his large house on the edge of the city.

On this particular day he was standing next to Elaine Wyllie, the headteacher, as they both watched a group of pupils taking a PE lesson inside the assembly hall. Wyllie takes up the story: 'Nigel turned to me and said: "Look at the children, Elaine, they're not fit!" I was a bit aghast, but on the other hand I could see what he meant. It was in part because he was from another era, wartime, when children were different.' Wyllie happened to mention the observation to the school's PE teacher, asking her if Buchanan was right. Wyllie recounts: 'She said: "I teach in five schools – only the fit ones are fit. Most of them are exhausted by the warmup in PE. The only exceptions are those in the running club, and girls and boys who play football. The rest? No, not fit."'

Soon afterwards Wyllie had to cover a PE lesson with a class of nine- and ten-year-olds. So she decided to see for herself: 'It was February, but it was mild, so I thought, "I know, I'll get them to run round the field as a warmup, and see how they get on." They were up for it, but it was like the polar opposite of *Chariots of Fire*. Five or six were in the running club and they were fine; they could have gone all day. But with the rest – it was a field the size of an ordinary football pitch, with a path round it, and most of them, by the far end of the field, were doubled up with a stitch, out of breath.'

Wyllie says she was appalled, but also, as she puts it, 'narked' at Buchanan for being right. So when the PE teacher returned they hatched a plan: get the class she had taught to run for fifteen minutes a day, every day, using a path around the same school field. They asked the pupils for ideas as to how this could work. One boy said his grandmother had got fit by running and walking alternately between lampposts on the streets, so they began by doing this, using the cherry trees on the route. And so it began. Wyllie says the idea was to review the programme in a month: 'I thought, "There'll be no review, this will fall apart."'

She was wrong. Most children were exhausted on the first couple of days. But by the end of the first week, she says, they were 'glowing', and appeared more focused in class. Soon, other classes wanted to take part, and before long the whole school was running every day. 'In that first month, the change in the children was transformational in terms of their fitness and their mental health,' she recalls. 'And in the following year or so, also in their body composition and their weight.'[1]

This was the beginning of the Daily Mile, a name which emerged by accident after the initial class wanted to know how far they were running. It turned out that the track was about a fifth of a mile long, and the pupils averaged five laps, with the distance staying broadly similar for every age group. Wyllie has since retired as a teacher and now leads a charity seeking to get the Daily Mile introduced into as many schools as possible. The energy giant Ineos sponsors the charity, and I meet her at their discreetly plush London offices, around the corner from Harrods.

For adults, running for fifteen minutes would very much be seen as formal exercise. But Wyllie stresses that this is not the case for children, particularly of primary age: 'We didn't try to introduce sport. It was just being active. It's about giving children, in a safe space, the opportunity to be children, and do what they do naturally.' The Daily Mile ethos, developed with the St Ninian's children in those initial few weeks, decrees that there is no special equipment or preparation needed. Children run in their school clothes, and it always takes place outside. It is meant to be sociable, so they can chat as they go. The running is non-competitive, allowing children to go at whatever pace they want, or even not at all, although Wyllie says the latter is rare: 'Very occasionally a child doesn't want to take part, and they stand aside for one minute, and then they start walking. And then they're running. It never fails.'

The aim is to be as inclusive as possible, with the lack of sports clothing avoiding any cultural or religious issues. Pupils with disabilities take part as well, with help if needed, and Wyllie says it has tended to prove very popular for children with autism. The Daily Mile is, she says, fifteen minutes of 'fun, fresh air, freedom, friends' in the school day: 'They very quickly get to the point of, "When's the Daily Mile?" It's not an escape from the classroom. Schools are much more child-pleasing than in my day. But they love and need the Daily Mile.'

It now takes place in over 7,000 primary schools around the UK, and has spread to more than seventy other countries. With this expansion has come new discoveries. Teachers can run as well if they want, and it has turned out this can provide a good moment for children to confide problems, whether about school or their home life.

Wylie says research has also shown that the Daily Mile is one of the few school-based interventions to defy a principle commonly seen in education called the 'Matthew effect'. This observes that if you start a programme aimed at assisting those who are least able, for example in reading, it often ends up widening the attainment gap because those who are already doing well improve even faster than the strugglers. But with the hugely steep dose–response curve for physical activity and health, the biggest gainers with the Daily Mile are children who began in the bottom 30 per cent for fitness levels.[2]

'All these things are happening because it's not sport, it's not PE – it's childhood,' Wyllie says. 'That was the key – children won't do what they don't like. They like it and that's why it's sustainable. I would not have given it a snowball's chance in you-know-where of succeeding. But even after that first month, we could see that we had stumbled on something. We knew it was sustainable, we knew it was universal and we knew it was transferable. A bit like ET coming to Elliott, the Daily Mile came to us. If Mr Buchanan had not said the children are not fit, I wouldn't be sitting here. It would never have happened. It was a completely serendipitous sentence, and good on him for having the cheek to say it.'

Wyllie is a hugely inspiring person to meet, and tells her story with genuine passion, even though I must be about the thousandth person to whom she has recounted it. And her scheme has achieved huge things. But in some ways, the Daily Mile is a symptom of failure. A typical ten-year-old should not be doubled up, wheezing, at the end of a few minutes' jog.

If the gradual evaporation of everyday activity is a worldwide crisis, then it is perhaps children who have been let down the most. Childhood, particularly in the pre-adolescence years of primary school, should be about constant movement – not sport, but self-guided exploration, exertion and fun. But for countless millions of modern children this is no longer the case.

There are many reasons why. A risk-averse culture has curtailed children's ability to roam under their own power. At the same time the dominance of motor traffic has created genuine peril to outdoor play, setting in place a vicious circle in which parents think the only way to keep their children safe is to drive them everywhere. Meanwhile in schools, ever-more intense academic curriculums have eroded time for play and sport, keeping children seated and docile during the moment in their lives when they should instead be at their most mobile, noisy and anarchic.

As we have seen, the UK statistics for adult inactivity are fairly bleak, with around a third of men and more than 40 per cent of women failing to meet even the minimum recommended level of 150 minutes of moderate activity per week.[3] For children the picture is considerably worse. When the last national study was completed in 2015, fewer than a quarter of children in England reached their required minimum of an hour a day of moderate-to-vigorous activity.[4] This is a global problem, with teenagers particularly at risk. As we saw in the first chapter, four in five adolescents worldwide are not sufficiently mobile, with almost all countries jeopardising their young people's future health.[5]

It is nonetheless a more complicated picture in some ways. For example, however adamant Nigel Buchanan was about the greater fitness of children from earlier generations, this can be difficult to prove definitively. Some research has disputed the idea of a long-term decline in children's aerobic capacity, or even that there is a definitive link between their physical activity levels and measurable fitness.

Other studies, however, side with Buchanan, and point to an apparently rapid physical decline. One research project assessed the aerobic fitness of ten- and eleven-year-olds in Essex in 2014 and compared it to tests done on the same age groups in 2008 and 1998. It found that a decline in fitness levels not only existed but was accelerating.[6] Another study, using data from the same group, found that while the children had become taller and heavier between 1998 and 2014, their muscular fitness was significantly lower.[7]

Direct comparisons with Buchanan's wartime-raised generation, let alone even earlier ones, is hugely difficult given a lack of directly comparable data. Some researchers have tried to get around that obstacle by studying modern youngsters who live in old-fashioned ways. Echoing the study of Amish farmers we saw earlier in the book, one group of Canadian researchers assessed the fitness of children from the Old Order Mennonites community, comparing them to their peers who live more typically modern lives. Like the Amish, the Mennonites reject all modern technologies, and the study found the children amassed about two or three hours a day of activity, mainly from walking and farm chores. Not unexpectedly, they tended to be leaner, stronger and fitter than the group living more contemporary lifestyles. One intriguing side note is that the only strength test in which the Mennonite children proved worse was press-ups. The researchers surmised that this was simply because they had never previously heard of a press-up, let alone tried to do one.[8]

Deficits in aerobic fitness and muscular strength can be fairly swiftly made up. As Elaine Wyllie discovered, the bodies of even habitually immobile children can be gratifyingly adaptable. But this cannot be put off forever. Movement in childhood is crucial to laying the groundwork for better overall health as an adult. Some of this can be linked to cardiovascular exertion. For example, one Danish study tested the fitness of about 750 nine-year-olds, and then examined them again ten years later. It found that even after accounting for other factors like allergies and heredity, the least fit children were four times more likely to have shown signs of asthma in the subsequent decade than the most fit.[9] While inactivity in itself does not cause asthma, for children with a risk of the condition, those with better fitness appear less likely to develop it.

Perhaps the most significant long-term impact is on bones. As we have seen in previous chapters, bones adapt to the repeated loads put on them, an effect officially known as Wolff's Law, after Julius Wolff, the nineteenth-century German anatomist who devised the theory. This plays a massive role in bone density, a key indicator of possible frailty in later life, notably through conditions like osteoporosis. About 70 per cent of the strength of our bones comes from their density.

A significant proportion of this is laid down in childhood, particularly adolescence, with bone density tending to peak in early adulthood. How much is laid down depends on the amount of force placed on the bones through physical motion. Studies have shown that the process known as healthy bone remodelling happens best between 2,000 and 4,000 microstrain units,[10] which translates into what should be the usual childhood regime of regular running, jumping and walking. This is especially vital for girls, who are more at risk from the consequences of weak bones when older. But this is not happening. Adolescence is precisely the moment when millions of children become less active, particularly girls. Teenage girls are not only less likely to be active than boys, but the gap is widening.

A huge World Health Organization study published in *The Lancet* in 2019 pulled together data from 146 countries to conclude that, worldwide, about 80 per cent of all children age eleven to seventeen are not sufficiently active. It found that over the previous fifteen years, while the proportion of inactive boys had actually fallen, from 80.1 per cent to 77.6 per cent, for girls it had remained steady at around 85 per cent – an activity gender gap of more than seven percentage points. Figures for the UK more or less exactly tracked this global trend.[11]

The reasons behind the low activity levels among teenagers, especially girls, are complex and long-standing, and often related, as we saw in Chapter 5, to a built environment geared more to the needs of boys. On a more cultural level, some of the best insights come from so-called qualitative studies, ones based not on raw data but exploring in detail people's motivations and reasons for certain behaviour. In 2000, England's now-defunct Health Education Authority produced a fascinating report using on in-depth interviews with children aged five to fifteen and their parents, which chronicled the influence of gender on activity as girls got older. 'I feel as if I don't want to stop,' one six-year-old girl is quoted as saying about her joy in running around. A bit later come the views of a pair of fifteen-year-old girls: 'Can't be bothered,' says one. 'Too much hard work,' adds her friend.[12] The reasons for the change were varied, but mainly connected to entrenched social attitudes, not least the pressures the teenage girls appeared to feel around fitting into gender stereotypes. An earlier study of young people in southeast London found similar attitudes. One fifteen-year-old girl said she and her friends had dropped out of playing school netball a couple of years earlier because they thought it was 'babyish'. This was a common attitude, the researchers found: 'Becoming a woman, according to the norms they had learned while growing up, usually meant that sport participation was given a low priority in their lives.'[13]

But it's not good enough to merely accept such views as inevitable. The authors of the 2019 WHO report into adolescent inactivity demanded urgent government action to address the situation, particularly for girls. 'Young people have the right to play and should be provided with the opportunities to realise their right to physical and mental health and wellbeing,' they said. 'That four in every five adolescents do not experience the enjoyment and social, physical, and mental health benefits of regular physical activity is not by chance, but a consequence of political choices and societal design.'[14]

Schools sitting down

A lot of these political choices manifest themselves inside schools, where children spend the bulk of their waking hours for five days a week during three quarters of the year. Many of the social and cultural norms they take into adulthood come from the classroom and playground. So what are our schools telling children about the importance of activity? It depends in part where you look.

As we will see in more detail in the next chapter, a handful of countries very deliberately try to ensure schools are places of constant activity. Finland has a long-standing programme called Finnish Schools on the Move, which is involved in everything from how children travel to school to the way they learn when they are there. How this happens is decided by teachers, but initiatives include longer break times to provide enough time for proper physical play, as well as learning based around movement, for example doing squats to count in maths classes. Students can stand in the classroom if they want, or sit on a ball. Another example is Slovenia, which has monitored the fitness of the nation's children for almost thirty years. Every school has two indoor sports areas and outside playgrounds and sports fields, plus access to government-owned nature camps converted from former military bases. Slovenia is now believed to be the only country in the world in which childhood obesity rates are falling.

In England, however, the centrally set curriculum does not even mandate any amount of physical education, even though it is a compulsory subject. A minimum of two hours per week is recommended, for both primary and secondary schools, but that is all it is – a recommendation.[15] A 2018 report found that around a third of English primary schools had less than this in their timetables.[16] The reasons vary, but it is often due to lack of time amid the increasingly long and arduous list of curriculum tasks which are compulsory, mainly formal academic work. There are valid reasons, particularly for primary schools, to focus on skills like language and maths as a way to even out the academic inequalities from differing home backgrounds. But many fear this has now subsumed thoughts of children's physical wellbeing.

In all Scottish schools, the two weekly hours of PE are compulsory,[17] even if, as shown by Elaine Wyllie's experience of her unfit nine- and ten-year-olds, this is generally not sufficient to counteract a lack of movement elsewhere in the children's lives. Wyllie told me that the packed schedule meant she initially doubted whether many other schools would take up even the fifteen minutes needed for the Daily Mile: 'It's an hour and a quarter a week out of a curriculum that's twenty-five hours long, and extremely precious.'

It is illustrative of the inertia towards activity in the wider

UK education system that despite the obvious success of the Daily Mile in her school, when Wyllie tried to get officials to pay attention she was initially met with suspicion: 'I couldn't get anybody interested. They should have been right at my door. Instead, I got my collar felt, because it was breaking the mould.' In the end, impetus built up for two reasons, Wyllie recalls: parents from neighbouring schools heard about the scheme and 'started to go to their headteacher and bash down the door'. Then, when St Ninian's started to win cross-country running events at a national level, even education authorities began paying attention.

The low status of physicality affects not just formal PE, but also classroom learning. While the youngest primary school pupils still spend much of their day sitting on carpets, before too long they are quietly writing at miniature tables, on their miniature chairs, like scale-model versions of the sedentary office workers so many will become. The amount of sitting involved in this, particularly as children get older, is the subject of considerable angst in the physical activity research world. One paper published in 2020 noted that in Australia, which despite its popular image as a land of bronzed sportspeople actually has a similar record on activity to the UK, pupils aged eight to twelve spent 60 per cent of their time in class sitting. 'Such broad attributes of classroom environments have changed little since the early 1900s,' the researchers noted.[18]

Equally important as healthy bones and well-developing cardiovascular systems, regular movement in childhood is vital as a template for future life. It is all the harder to persuade an adult they should cycle into work, or sit less over the day, if all they have known is cars and chairs.

My nine-year-old son goes to a state primary school which in many ways is admirable. The teachers are committed and hugely hardworking, and they genuinely care about their young charges. It has made real efforts to get more children walking and cycling to school, blocking off the street at drop-off and pick-off times. But I worry whether it has quite got the message on physical movement during learning hours. It has yet to sign up to the Daily Mile, even if in fairness, as a cramped London school whose only grass playing field is occasionally borrowed from the very expensive private school next door, this could be for logistical reasons. Before his formal school year was curtailed by the coronavirus lockdown, it was not uncommon for my son to recount that PE was cancelled to make room for some other part of school life, often to catch up with academic obligations. It was noticeable that he would sometimes get out of school at 3:30pm seeming a bit pent-up and restless.

So I decided to enlist him for a brief, if surreptitious, experiment. With his consent – in fact he was very keen on the idea – he spent an entire school day shortly before lockdown wearing the tiny Danish-made activity tracker I had used to monitor my own sitting time for the last chapter, carefully taped to his thigh underneath his school trousers. For comparison, he then wore the tracker the following Saturday.

If you have not had much recent experience of nine-year-old boys, their default setting when left to their own devices is to be in motion, or at least standing. More or less the only exceptions are watching a screen, reading, or mealtimes. Even these are not a given. When eating his breakfast my son's preferred habit is to place his cereal bowl on the living room windowsill and eat standing up, flicking through a football magazine.

After I download the data from his days wearing the activity tracker, the readings for the Saturday reflect this way of life. The chart, plotting the day in fifteen-minute chunks, is more or less entirely filled in with the orange, yellow and blue lines to show walking, sporadic walking and standing, even if there is a break to show that, apparently, this was one of the days when he decided to eat breakfast sitting down. The movement is not all spontaneous. There is a splash of bright green lines to show running in the mid-morning, when he was doing his usual Saturday tennis lesson with friends in our local park. But with the time in bed factored out over the 24-hour period, the accumulated inactive time comes to little more than two hours.

When I first look at the chart for his day at school, the contrast is immediate, and dispiriting. Before school and after is the same as the Saturday – a mass of colour to show movement. But from 9am to 3:30pm the backdrop is mainly the drab grey that indicates sitting. It is not unbroken. There are bursts of activity, particularly at breaktime and during lunch. But between that, the bulk of the day is clearly spent in a chair. In both the morning and afternoon there are two-hour periods where the inactivity is barely interrupted at all. The combined total for daytime sitting is more than six hours – three times as much as the weekend.

As we saw in the last chapter, excessive sitting can mark the start of a gradual pathway towards type 2 diabetes and obesity. For a minority of children the former is not even that far in the future. Type 2 diabetes was always seen as a condition of middle age and later. We saw in Chapter 4 how there are now more than 7,000 under-25s in England and Wales recorded as having the condition. Almost unbelievably, some of them are still in school, even primary school.[19]

I'm not a teacher, and I can only try to imagine the difficulties of corralling a class of thirty children to make sure they all learn to the best of their abilities, and how much easier that must be if they are sitting down. But if we ever want our children to grow up healthy, active and delighted with their own, in-built, everyday thirst for movement, this is not how you do it.

A life of confinement

There is, of course, much more to the issue than sitting in school. There has been considerable public hand wringing in recent years about the perceived cosseting of children, with a lack of independence meaning many are ferried more or less everywhere in a parent's car. Physical play is supervised and limited, without previous generations' ability to roam, explore and experiment.

These worries are based in fact. A useful indicator for independent childhood mobility is how children get to and from school, and there is no doubt the statistics show a decline in active travel. In England, more than four in ten primary pupils are taken to school in a car, even though many of these trips are under a mile.[20] Australia keeps particularly detailed figures on school travel. One study found that in 1971, 58 per cent of schoolchildren aged nine or younger in Sydney would walk to school, with 23 per cent driven. Thirty years later the figures were 26 per cent walking and 67 per cent in cars.[21]

What is the difference? Again, the villain of the piece is towns and cities dominated by motor traffic. Fear of road danger by parents is both obvious and understandable. Globally, road injuries are the leading cause of death among children and young people, killing more than AIDS, tuberculosis and diseases like dysentery, combined.[22] In the UK, 70 per cent of parents who drive their primary-age children to school cite danger from cars as the main reason, even as their own transport choice adds to the problem.[23] This does not only rob children of mobility. It also takes away their freedom to move about without relying on their parents.

And yet, at least in the UK, statistics seem to show the roads are getting notably safer. In 1930, despite vastly lower numbers of motor vehicles, 1,685 child pedestrians were killed.[24] As recently as 2001 there were 219 child road deaths.[25] In 2018, the most current data, there were forty-eight.[26] Given this astonishing safety increase, why is everyone so scared? One reason, of course, is that travel decisions are based on perceived danger, and not statistics. But there is another theory.

In 1990, Mayer Hillman, a radical architect-turned-campaigner for liveable cities, published a study into childhood independence and mobility, the message of which still resonates today. It was called *One False Move*, the title taken from a then-current government-run traffic safety campaign showing a child about to step off a kerb into the road, with the slogan, 'One false move and you're dead.' Hillman sought to understand the reasons for such scare tactics when, even at that point, the government was boasting with some justification about how much safer the roads had become, with deaths having fallen by a third since the 1960s. The police, he noted, had declared the UK's roads the safest in Europe. What was going on?

The think tank Hillman worked with, the Policy Studies Institute, had carried out a series of surveys in 1971 in five areas of England about children's independence and mobility. He decided to replicate these, and the findings were striking. For example, in 1971, more than 80 per cent of eight-year-olds were allowed to go to school unaccompanied. Less than twenty years later this had fallen to about 10 per cent. The proportion of all children allowed to ride their bike on the road fell from nearly 70 per cent to 25 per cent. The same picture emerged in virtually every aspect of the children's active lives.

Hillman quoted the writer Roald Dahl recounting his joy as a six-year-old in 1922 racing his sister on his tricycle on the near-deserted roads where he grew up in Wales. The further back you went, Hillman noted, the greater the likelihood of an adult recalling the 'good old days' of such an independent, mobile childhood. Modern children, he argued, were not any safer; they were just more confined. 'The "good old days" of reminiscence and the "good new days" depicted by the accident statistics are reconciled by the loss of children's freedom,' Hillman said. 'The streets have not become safer, they have become, as the government's poster proclaims, extremely dangerous. It is the response to this danger, by both children and their parents, that has contained the road accident death rate.'[27] This is a vital point, and one ministers are understandably coy about when discussing traffic casualties. Childhood might now be safer, particularly on the roads, but when this is mainly achieved by shutting young people in their homes, this is something of a pyrrhic victory.

Of course, if Hillman were to carry out the studies for a third time, the restrictions on children's mobility would be significantly greater even than in 1990. None of this is to blame parents, just to acknowledge that instilling activity into children is severely hampered by the way our towns, cities and roads are designed. This matters because activity habits in one part of children's lives tend to spill over into another. A study by Scottish academics which fitted activity trackers to a group of thirteen- and fourteen-year-olds in Edinburgh found that those who walked to school also racked up significantly more moderate and vigorous physical activity in their leisure time than those who were driven, and even compared to those who took the train or bus.[28]

Tim Gill, the campaigner and adviser on mobility and play, whom we first heard from in Chapter 5, has spent many years warning governments, generally in vain, that the priorities of modern life are having a hugely disadvantageous effect on children's health and wellbeing. 'It's very clear that children are out and playing less, pretty much all over the world,' he says. 'And it's also clear that the design of residential neighbourhoods, especially, is a key reason for that. There's hard evidence that both the speed and volume of traffic leads kids to be outdoors less. If you take a sort of historical view, you could almost say that the story of children and urban areas over the twentieth century was about the battle between children and cars. And in simple terms the children lost.'

Gill notes that this phenomenon has seen the play enjoyed by children not just reducing, but becoming more structured and formalised. With cars banishing young people from the streets, they were obliged to use playgrounds and other artificial spaces. 'The history of playgrounds is that they first emerged in cities as a response to traffic,' he says. 'So 150 years ago, during industrialization and the first wave of urbanisation, kids played in the street. But when cars started appearing, people started saying: this isn't going to work. But kids still needed somewhere to play, so they created playgrounds.'[29]

Gill has written a book, *No Fear: Growing Up in a Risk-Averse Society*, which argues that beyond even cars, the modern world has become both fearful and mistrustful of children doing very ordinary childhood things. He cites a case in the West Midlands in which three twelve-year-olds were arrested and had DNA samples taken for climbing a cherry tree which was on public land, which police justified on the basis of antisocial behaviour.

Children, Gill argues, need to be not only physically active, but sometimes active in an environment that includes risk, and has not had all the dangers, glitches and uncertainties designed out in advance by adults. He uses this resonant quote from Helle Nebelong, a Danish landscape architect who specialises in natural play spaces: 'When the distance between all the rungs in a climbing net or a ladder is exactly the same, the child has no need to concentrate on where he puts his feet. Standardisation is dangerous because play becomes simplified and the child does not have to worry about his movements. This lesson cannot be carried over to all the knobbly and asymmetrical forms with which one is confronted throughout life.'[30]

This, as much as anything, is the choice we make by confining children to brief, supervised trips to playgrounds, or otherwise cocooning them inside vehicles, and quietening them at school desks. Such things become habituated into adulthood. This is not to blame parents, or teachers. As with every discussion of everyday activity, the one about the increasingly passive, inert, regularised nature of modern childhoods cannot be seen outside the physical and educational environment in which they take place. But when it comes to future health, or even the chance to appreciate the everyday bliss of regular exertion, our children are being badly let down.

Ageing as a project

One of the overriding themes of this book has been the idea that for physical activity to truly stick in the mass of people's lives, it has to be integrated, or incidental, to use the public health term – part of someone's daily routine, not a hard-to-schedule leisure activity. And yet, as research for this chapter, I find myself in a local gym, being led through an introductory session of stretches, squats and assorted weightlifting. What's going on?

This is the moment where I introduce the one slight exception to the part-of-everyday-life mantra: staying active in older age. Of course, there are people in their sixties, seventies or older who acquire their daily dose of movement as they go about their business, for example cycling and walking around, or gardening. But for many people, this simply does not happen, not least because regular active travel is often tied to a commute. However, one advantage enjoyed by many older people is more time. That is why many experts on activity and ageing advise people to, in effect, see healthy ageing as a project – not a job, but certainly important enough to set aside time for every week. When people retire, they need to construct a new schedule for their days based around something other than the workplace. As part of this, the guidance goes, why not include some formal exercise?

This advice is not, however, getting across. If mass inactivity in children heralds a looming health crisis for the future, among the ever-growing population of older people worldwide this emergency has well and truly arrived. The UK has some of the most thorough age-based statistics for inactivity, and they make for alarming reading. Across all ages, 62 per cent of adults meet the minimum activity recommendations, and as you might expect, is it higher in young people, reaching 72 per cent for the under-35s. But the decline with age is steep. For people in their mid-fifties, 57 per cent are sufficiently active, and by sixty-five this falls to 55 per cent. Among those seventy-five plus, fewer than a third manage the minimum, and over half are totally inactive.[31] It is a similar pattern for sedentariness, with official estimates saying those aged sixty-five and over spend an average of ten hours sitting down each day.[32]

There is an extent to which your reaction might be: well, so what? Older people do become more infirm, and have less energy. Many people, if they think of a grandparent, will conjure up a mental image of someone sitting in an overstuffed armchair with a cup of tea. If someone is retired, don't they deserve a bit of a rest?

It's not that simple. In modern terms, sixty-five is now simply not that old. UK life expectancy from birth is over eighty,[33] and there are around 600,000 people aged ninety or older, a population which grows every year.[34] But as we saw in Chapter 4, the gap between life expectancy and the age when the average person suffers some sort of impairment is now almost twenty-one years for women, and over sixteen years for men.[35] Medical advances are helping to extend life expectancy across the globe, but these extra years come at a cost. Some studies have suggested that, for the average person in a country like the UK or US, 40 per cent of any additional time gained will simply be spent in a care home.[36] This is not something countries can afford. But just as importantly, it's really not something anyone as an individual wants to go through.

This crisis is approaching on two fronts. People are becoming immobile and sedentary at increasingly younger ages, meaning they are ever more likely to arrive in their sixties or seventies already struggling with one or more of the conditions linked to inactivity, most notably type 2 diabetes or poor cardiovascular function. But also, as people get older they tend to move even less, exacerbating existing conditions.

Part of this is down to a lack of aerobic exertion. Activity guidelines for older people are the same as for other adults – at a minimum, they should aim for 150 minutes of moderate activity a week, or half that amount if it is vigorous.[37] But as people age the other, often-neglected aspect of the activity guidelines becomes increasingly vital – muscle strengthening. The gradual wastage of muscle mass as someone gets older, known as sarcopenia, can significantly affect their ability to live independently. Older people can lose up to 40 per cent of their muscle mass.[38] However, this is by no means inevitable, and is likely to be a consequence of long-term lack of use as much as advancing years. In fact, so strong are similarities between the changes associated with inactivity and those seen with ageing, notably muscle wastage, that some researchers have theorised that to an extent we are mistaking the former for the latter, and that much age-related decline is simply down to long-term bodily underuse.

Numerous studies have shown that weight-based training can improve not just strength, but also balance, making falls less likely. It can also help slow down reductions in bone density, another key factor for a thriving older age. It has additionally been shown to help with arthritis, the often crippling condition of joint pain and inflammation, which affects around one in five Britons from middle age and onwards.[39] Thus, more or less every activity advice for older people now generally recommends some sort of strength training at least twice a week, with the US guidelines in particular saying these should 'involve all major muscle groups'.[40] Along with this is advice to work on balance and flexibility. The official NHS guidelines list examples of strength exercises as carrying heavy shopping bags, or vigorous gardening chores such as digging.[41]

However, not everyone lives within walking distance of the shops, or has a garden. This is where strength-based formal exercise can come in. It can involve something as simple as press-ups and sit-ups, or activities which combine strength and flexibility, for example yoga and Pilates. Another option is to go to a gym. For all that these can remain intimidating places, an increasing number have tried to become more welcoming for older people, and have staff and equipment which make resistance training very different from the stereotype of sweaty, bulky men clanging iron weights.

And so it was I found myself in my local gym. I am still some way off both retirement and the full onset of potential muscle wastage, but I put myself forward as a sort of underaged guinea pig, asking the local gym if they could imagine I was a sixty-plus customer and demonstrate to me the sort of regime I would be put through. In the basement of a local library, the gym is run by a non-profit social enterprise called Better, who operate a series of leisure centres across London. They have a particular specialism in what they call active ageing, and organise an annual 'Over-55s Olympics', in which various gyms in the chain compete against each other.

Alistair Imbeah, the hugely enthusiastic and reassuring instructor who takes me for my example session, tells me he works with a lot of older gym-goers, both individually and in classes. My most abiding impression is that if, as he claims, mine is the sort of routine most sixty-pluses would expect, his customers must be a pretty fit bunch. Imbeah leads me through an initial callisthenics-based workout of planks and squats which leaves even my cycling-trained legs feeling it by the end.

But the most eye-opening part is when we move onto the weights. The room does have the usual array of resistance machines and shiny metal barbells racked in ascending size. But he uses softer, much less intimidating weights, mainly soft and padded, which wouldn't hurt too much if you dropped them on your foot. These include weighted pouches without handles, which are designed to also help improve hand grip, another area which often deteriorates with age. It's challenging, and I ache a bit the next day, but no one could realistically call it intimidating.

Never too late

For all that some people do embrace gym-going or other forms of activity and exercise in later life, there are plenty who quietly conclude that after decades of immobility, there might not be much point. This could not be more wrong. There is, seemingly, never an age point at which regular exertion does not bring benefits. Countless studies have shown that, even among notably old-age test subjects, programmes of aerobic or resistance activities, or both, coupled with balance and flexibility work, can not just slow the gradual decline caused by the advancing years but reverse it, making continued independent living all the more likely.

At the more unusual end of this, some people take up activity in middle age or beyond, and suddenly find they are actually very good at it. As we saw in Chapter 3, Ralph Paffenbarger only started running well into his forties, but before too long was completing marathons in under three hours. Perhaps my favourite example of a late-starter is John Keston, a relatively little-known English actor and singer who settled in the US after appearing on Broadway with the Royal Shakespeare Company. While he never achieved much fame on the stage, he did make something of a name for his extraordinary late-life athletic achievements. In his mid-fifties, and with no sporting experience to speak of, Keston decided to try a couple of fun runs to combat high blood pressure. He turned out to be not only an excellent runner, but one seemingly undaunted by age. At seventy he missed out by less than a minute on becoming the first-ever runner from that age group to beat three hours in a marathon, and set dozens of veterans records.[42] Last heard of, three years ago, aged ninety-two, he was still running four times a week, covering several miles at a time.[43]

The good news is that you don't have to be running marathons, let alone in under or close to three hours, to feel the health benefits of latter-age activity. It's worth remembering that in terms of exertion, moderate and vigorous are relative terms, and as you age the amount needed to push your body into the magic zone beyond three METs necessarily becomes less. As we saw in Chapter 2 with the health gains acquired by the American over-seventies from even a few thousand fairly sedate daily steps, there is emerging evidence that in older age relatively tiny amounts of movement can do a lot of good.

And this is not just about physical welfare. It is also true for what many activity experts consider perhaps the most exciting and fast-moving area of activity research: the mounting evidence that regular movement can ward off Alzheimer's and other forms of dementia, as well as giving an overall boost to cognitive function. Some studies have even shown that it can reverse the shrinking of the brain that otherwise happens as we age.

Kirk Erickson, a professor of psychology at the University of Pittsburgh and one of the world's foremost experts in how activity can help the ageing brain, tells me: 'We think that starting earlier in life is probably better, as is the way for most things. But that doesn't mean it's ever too late to start. And that's an important message. Some people that come into my studies say, "Well, I've never exercised in my life, it's probably too late for me." And I like to tell them that it's never too late. It's a shame that sometimes people start thinking that they're on an inevitable trajectory, and there's nothing they can do.'[44]

One thing that is abundantly clear from dozens of studies is that the more active and fit someone is in older age, the better their chances of living even longer. We have already seen that activity has been shown to seemingly slow the ageing process by limiting the shortening of telomeres, the end-caps for our chromosomes. The study we saw before estimated the benefit at around nine years. Others have gone higher – one UK research paper said the most inactive of a group who had their telomere length measured 'may be biologically older by ten years compared with more active subjects'.[45]

One US study that examined the fitness of more than 4,000

sixty-pluses found, a dozen years later, that those in the upper 40 per cent of tested fitness were around half as likely to have died as those in the bottom 20 per cent.[46] An even longer-term study, over twenty-one years, found that 15 per cent of older members from a California running club died over that period, against 34 per cent of same-age non-runners. Even more strikingly, when age-related disability was measured, while it took the non-runners just 2.6 years on average to start finding some everyday tasks difficult, for the runners it was 8.7 years.[47] It's worth remembering that this is about lifelong fitness, not just a previous history of activity – exertion must be maintained and regular for its benefits to be felt.

A decline in independent living can take many forms, and can be mental as well as physical. One UK study which tried to project the future scope of so-called multi-morbidity – the prevalence of a series of chronic conditions in one person – found that in 2015, more than half of Britons aged sixty-five and over had two or more conditions from a list including arthritis and high blood pressure – the two most common – as well as diabetes, cancer and dementia. By 2025 this proportion was expected to increase to almost two thirds.[48]

Another crucial factor is bone strength, particularly for women, whose bone density diminishes after the menopause. Osteoporosis, the chronic condition caused by low bone density, is one of the major causes of impairment, and often death, in older people, causing an estimated 9 million fractures a year worldwide. Osteoporosis groups say the condition affects 10 per cent of women in their sixties, 20 per cent of those in their seventies, and 40 per cent of those in their eighties.[49]

But while, as we saw earlier, a considerable proportion of bone density is laid down in youth, it is once again never too late to start. Numerous studies have shown that activity can halt or even reverse the age-related decay of bones, and make fractures less likely. Part of the picture is also preventing falls in the first place, which is a function also of strength and balance, hence the importance of muscular training.

Professor David Buchner from the University of Illinois is one of the world's best-known experts on inactivity science. He spent nine years in charge of physical activity for the US Centers for Disease Control and Prevention, and chaired the group that wrote the American government's first official guidelines on the subject. Much of his recent work has been connected to how strength-based activity and balance exercises can prevent falls in older people.

'It is amazing,' he says. 'I mean, an older adult can reduce the risk of a fracture by 40 per cent by doing these balance exercises and lumbar strength training. We're not talking training Olympic athletes here, we're talking about fairly modest, moderate amounts of physical activity on a regular basis. And it has that level of effect on older adults.'[50]

Scores out of ten

Because healthy ageing takes in so many elements – aerobic fitness, muscular strength, balance, flexibility, a lack of chronic impairment – it can sometimes be hard to measure without medical expertise. But there are shortcuts. Perhaps the best-known is usually called the sit–stand test, otherwise known as the chair test. Largely assessing muscular power and endurance, as well as elements of balance, this begins with the subject sitting upright on a straight-backed, non-padded chair without arm rests, with their feet flat on the floor and arms folded with the hands on each opposite shoulder. They must then rise, unaided, to a full stand and sit down again as many times as possible within thirty seconds.

Men aged sixty to sixty-four should be able to manage around fourteen, and women twelve, with the recommended minimum gradually decreasing as people age more. Below-average scores have been linked in studies with a greater likelihood of death, as well as more chance of falling.[51]

There are other tests which studies have shown to be good indicators of longevity, for example grip strength. Another gauge, demonstrated by a 2014 UK study and more recently popularised by Michael Mosley, the TV doctor and media sage on better ageing, is whether or not someone can stand on one foot for thirty seconds with their eyes closed.[52] This is based on the importance of balance as we get older, and the connection between poor balance and possible later dementia.

Perhaps the most thorough and ingenious, if less well known, is a distant variant of the chair test devised by a Brazilian doctor called Claudio Gil Araujo, who runs a clinic in Rio and has focused on sports and exercise since the 1970s. Araujo says he became fascinated with the idea of discovering a tell-all test for older patients after noting that some of them, for example runners, were aerobically fit but had poor flexibility, or limited all-body muscular strength.

With the help of his wife, who has a doctorate in physical education, Araujo devised what is called the sit–rise test. This is marginally more complex to explain than the chair test, but even easier to do at home. All it needs is a flat, non-slippery space of about two metres square. The person being tested stands in the middle of this, barefoot, and wearing clothing that won't restrict their movements. They are then given the deceptively simple instruction: 'Without worrying about the speed of movement, try to sit and then to rise from the floor, using the minimum support that you believe is needed.'

The aim is to do this without using your hands, either on the floor or on a knee. It's permitted to cross your legs if you want, but you cannot then rise by using the sides of your feet as a lever – they must be flat as you stand up. You are then scored out of ten, five each for the sit and the rise. A point is taken off for any support used, with half a point deducted for unsteadiness or loss of balance.

It sounds straightforward, and in many ways it is. But the beauty of the sit–rise test is the number of elements it examines in one go. To score a ten you need not just good flexibility and balance, but also both strength and power in your muscles. These are different traits. Strength is simply the ability of your body to produce enough force to move something, whether your own body or an external object; power is about producing the greatest amount of force in the shortest possible time, and is seen as particularly important for healthy ageing.

Speaking from his clinic in Rio, Araujo tells me that when he started to use the test he discovered it also, indirectly, measured other risk factors: 'We perceived that if you ask someone to sit on the floor and rise from the floor, we are evaluating at the same time several things, including body composition. Because if you are overweight, you have problems sitting normally on the floor and even more problems with rising from the floor.'[53]

Araujo's clinic has an easily searchable YouTube video[54] showing how the test should be done. But be warned, it can be addictive. If you give the instructions to a child they will inevitably drop lightly to the floor, and rise again without apparent effort – indeed, it is seen as a worry if someone under eighteen cannot manage this manoeuvre with the full ten points. But as people age, the various infirmities begin to take effect.

For example, I like to think I can manage a safe ten, although a particularly strict marker might occasionally dock me half a point for lack of grace on the descent. But even while I manage this, the sit–rise test betrays where my score is likely to decline with age. As someone who cycles a fair bit, I have fairly strong legs for my weight, particularly in the quadriceps, the large muscles at the front of your thighs which you also use a lot to stand up. Sadly, also like a lot of people who ride a bike, I also don't stretch nearly enough, and the flexibility in my legs and hips is gradually diminishing. I can still rise from the floor without support, but I'm aware that this is largely the power in my legs overcoming the lack of movement. It's a trick I won't be able to pull off forever, unless I start working on my flexibility. I have been warned.

Araujo argues that his creation is more effective than the chair test, in part because it gauges so many elements, but also because it avoids any equipment skewing the results, for example differing relative heights of people and the chair they use. "We found one way to have a sort of a simple score that everybody can understand,' Araujo says. 'As a physician, many times my patients would come to me and say, "Doctor, what do these lab results mean?" This tells them.'

There is, however, more to it than a score out of ten. Araujo devised the test in the late 1990s, just to use with his older patients. But some years later a visiting US academic suggested Araujo compare the score with mortality records. He worked with postgraduate students to do this, and they found a striking link – the lower someone's sit–rise score, the more likely they were to die. 'Those who have a score of zero to two or three – they have really bad chances of surviving compared to those who have eight to ten,' he says.

The first tranche of results found that among the 200 or so people who scored zero in the test, meaning they needed help to sit or stand, the death rate was 4.3 per cent a year on average, odds as bad as some forms of cancer. In contrast, of the 480 of his patients who scored from eight to ten, only four died over the eight-year study period, despite being aged between forty and eighty.[55] 'These are just ordinary people. We're not looking for anyone from the circus or anything,' Araujo says. His oldest-ever scorer of a ten was aged seventy-three. Araujo, who is sixty-four but a keen runner, manages 8.5, shedding half a point for a wobble on the way down, and a full point for using one hand to rise. This still puts him in the 90th score percentile for his age group, he tells me proudly.

Growing your brain

Physical prowess is only half the battle when it comes to vibrant, independent ageing. Dementia, notably Alzheimer's, is one of the most common reasons for older people needing outside care. The idea that activity could not just slow this decline, but to an extent rewind it, has obvious individual benefits. On a population-wide level, however, the implications are astounding. Amid fast-ageing populations, there are an estimated 10 million new cases of dementia worldwide every year.[56] In the UK there are currently 850,000 people living with dementia, with the total cost of care exceeding £30 billion.[57] By 2040, both figures are forecast to have doubled. Tackling this alone would seem sufficient justification for just about any government to start intervening to make life-time physical activity more common.

If prompted, most people probably know that mental stimulation, particularly into older age, is known to reduce the risk of dementia and other forms of cognitive decline. But the fact that this is also true of physical activity remains far less understood, despite several decades of studies on the subject. Research in this area has rocketed with the advent of brain-scanning technologies which allow scientists to not just test the changes prompted by physical exertion, but observe them.

Kirk Erickson, who has led a series of these studies, is clear about the weight of evidence. 'We can be very confident that greater amounts of physical activity reduce your risk of developing Alzheimer's. That is something I am wholeheartedly confident of saying,' he tells me. 'I would also say that the evidence is very strong that engaging in moderate amounts of physical activity is beneficial for brain cognitive function.'[58]

The latter area is one of the most fascinating areas of current research. Among studies Erickson has led includes ones which used randomised trials to show aerobic exercise both improved memory and actually increased the size of the hippocampus, a part of the brain connected to both memory and the mental complex tasks known as executive functions.[59]

Erickson explains what these are: 'For an example, your ability right now to selectively attend to what I'm saying and ignore distracting information, that's considered a component of executive function. Your ability to maintain items in working memory for short periods of time, and work on that material, that's also considered executive function. Your ability to switch between doing different tasks, between, you know, typing an email, and then jumping in and finishing up a document and then jumping back, maybe in a work environment, that's also executive function.'

Such tasks, of course, are central to maintaining an independent life. 'Absolutely,' Erickson says. 'Unfortunately it's one of the areas of cognitive function that shows some early losses. So if we're able to improve executive function with modest amounts of regular physical activity, that is very important.' Regular activity has been shown to at least mitigate such losses, but can even prompt improvements – up to a certain point. Erickson adds: 'One caveat is that it is a moderate-sized effect, which means that you're not going to be jumping several IQ points just by doing exercise.'

This effect is, of course, particularly beneficial for people at risk of dementia, which is generally characterised by memory loss and a decline in higher cognitive abilities. One study took a group of older people in Australia who had the beginnings of memory problems but had not reached the threshold for Alzheimer's. Half were randomly allocated a six-month regime of physical activity, with the others given a programme of education on ageing. At the end of this period the physical group showed some improvements on the scale to test for Alzheimer's, while the others saw a clearly measurable decline.[60] As with many elements of physical activity in older age, the key appears to be to do at least something physical, and perhaps worrying less about whether it is sufficiently strenuous or specialised. For example, in the just-mentioned Alzheimer's research, the most common type of activity for the group who saw the improvement was simply walking.

This is still a relatively new area, and Erickson says that when he began doing studies he faced widespread scepticism that something so simple, and without the need for any drugs, could be effective in combating dementia. 'In recent years I think the tide is changing,' he says. 'We're now at a point where the wealth of data that we have can no longer really be ignored. And then there's the cost of pharmaceuticals and the failure of pharmaceuticals to really prevent and treat many neurologic conditions. When I go to meetings, sometimes pharmaceutical representatives will stand up and discuss the failures of their trials, and they'll even be in favour of more work being done examining the impact of these types of behavioural modifications.'

This is a hugely powerful idea, and one that again ties in with the conceit of this book's title. In being active, at any age, we might not be literally ingesting a tablet, but its effect on our bodies is to help them create a bespoke internal cocktail that can reduce the risk of disease, improve our strength, endurance, balance and power, not to mention even increase the size and function of our brain. It's perhaps no wonder the pharmaceutical companies are starting to realise they can't compete.

Next steps:

If you have children, even if it does feel like they are always sprinting around at home, think about how active they actually are, and whether they are meeting the hour-a-day recommended movement – or three hours a day for younger children. And if you are older, don't forget the importance of balance, as well as strength and aerobic fitness, for healthy ageing.

9

The Power of Social Engineering

It is shortly after 9am, the temperature is –13°C, and a light snow
is falling. Even though I am heavily wrapped in several layers
of clothing, including long johns, a thick skiing jacket and two
hats, my teeth have begun to chatter. But in front of me, on a
school playground covered in several weeks' worth of thickly
encrusted snow, something fairly unlikely is happening: several
dozen children are cycling around.

I am in Joensuu, a small city in northeast Finland, about 250
miles from Helsinki and only a few dozen miles from the Russian
border, which has the slightly niche claim of being one of the
winter cycling capitals of the world. Despite undeniably brutal
winters – on the February evening when I arrive on the train
from Helsinki, Finland's capital city, it is –16°C, and the mercury
never goes above –6°C when I am there – about 20 per cent of all
journeys in the city are made by bike.[1] This is a year-round average
and in winter the figure does understandably fall somewhat. Even
so, during my visit, cyclists are still a routine sight, crunching
serenely along the cycle paths, or at least what I presume are cycle
paths hidden underneath the several inches of flattened snow.

If you set aside the weather, Joensuu has several advantages for cycling, including that it is almost entirely flat. It is also geographically compact, with about three quarters of the 80,000 population living within a gentle twenty-minute bike ride of the centre. Many locals are young, with about 10 per cent being students. Finally, much of the city is new – as recently as the 1950s the population was only 7,000 – and so the streets are wide, with plenty of space for cycle lanes.

But its friendliness for year-round cycling is no accident. As Juha-Pekka Vartiainen, who is in charge of road infrastructure for the city council, tells me: 'There's a long tradition of cycling here. But we also have a long tradition of planning for cycling.'[2] This includes many years of constructing safe bike routes away from the motor traffic, whether entirely separated lanes or the shared use of a wide pavement. As Vartiainen points out, bike lanes simply painted onto the road will not work in a city where they would be invisible below the snow for several months a year. The bike routes are also, like the roads, ploughed after every new snowfall. Rather than scraping back to the tarmac, the ploughs smooth the snow flat, adding grooves for extra traction. This might sound counterintuitive, but as long as the temperature remains below freezing, it creates a remarkably grippy surface, and the bulk of Joensuu's cyclists ride with normal tyres, not the metal-studded winter type seen in many other similarly freezing cities.

But there is another, hugely important, factor in play. This is not just a regional quirk; year-round physical activity, and the many ways to create it, is a major priority of Finland's national government. In the case of the primary school I visit, about a quarter of pupils cycle year-round, teachers tell me. Admittedly, their numbers are probably greater than normal on this particular morning. An instructor from Helsinki has arrived, and he is leading the students through snow-cycle training and a series of games, including an obstacle course and a contest in which two teams try to move a cardboard box by cycling past and hitting it with snowballs.

This is the opening event of something called the Winter Cycling Congress, which brings together politicians, officials and experts to share information on year-round riding. Pitching up in a different chilly location every year, the Congress is a proudly low-budget event, run by a committee of volunteers and reliant on host cities to provide a venue. But this time, things are a bit more lavish than normal. As well as a generous event space, inside a vast, wood-built indoor sports arena adjoining one of the city's universities, there are tours, excursions, and a drinks reception at Joensuu's art gallery, hosted by the mayor. Finland's central government has underwritten most costs, including the flights and accommodation for many attendees and media, me among them. Why? It is because physical activity is something the country takes very, very seriously, and it would like the world to know about this.

A couple of days before arriving in Joensuu I head to Finland's 1920s parliament building, an austere, classical-meets-modernist stone structure which looms across the centre of Helsinki. I am meeting Krista Kiuru, Finland's minister for family affairs and social services, whose brief covers preventative health. She is, incidentally, among a majority of female ministers in a government led by Sanna Marin, who was just thirty-four when she became prime minister.

Kiuru makes a fascinating argument for why the Finnish government is so keen on pushing everyday physical activity: as with the country's famously excellent and much-studied education system, she says, it is not just of obvious benefit to citizens but can act as an international beacon for a small and not hugely powerful country of just over 5 million people.

'It's a basic value here in Finland that we encourage our citizens to be active in life. It is kind of a way to see that if Finland's people can be active, then we can be better as a nation,' Kiuru tells me during our lengthy chat in parliament, a conversation periodically interrupted by aides reminding her, in vain, that she is running late for her next engagement.

'We're not rich in natural resources. There's no oil. But what we can do is similar to what we have done with schools, which is a very well-known product around the world. It is the same here. When we talk about the health system, we're talking about the equal right to have good services. We encourage everyone to be active, to be as healthy as possible. It's the same way we're encouraging the pupils in the schools to do their best, to be as good as their potential.'[3]

This is inspiring stuff. And there is little doubt that by most international standards, Finland is generally a success story when it comes to an active population. In the awkwardly named Eurobarometer surveys, huge EU-wide polls on many areas of life across the member states, Finland routinely has the highest proportion of people who say they take part in at least some sport or exercise, currently at 87 per cent. The UK equivalent is 63 per cent, which is actually above average – at the bottom sits Bulgaria, where fewer than a third of people ever do any formal exercise. Finland is also near the top for the EU rankings for non-sport physical activity, although it is beaten by the Netherlands and Denmark, both helped by their very high levels of everyday cycling.[4]

The Dutch and Danish levels of bike use are, of course, a product of decades of central government-led policy and spending decisions to boost active travel. This is the sort of thing which to many British politicians' eyes would cross into the territory of social engineering. But it is worth remembering that much of the impetus for these changes came from the public. We saw earlier that the transport revolution in the Netherlands was sparked by the *Stop de Kindermoord* (Stop the Child Murders) road safety mass protests of the 1970s. Copenhagen saw similar scenes later in that decade and into the 1980s, pushing authorities into action.

In contrast, the transformation of Finland's public health was even more dramatic, but was also a notably top-down, almost paternalistic enterprise, led by scientists and researchers who enlisted the help of politicians to persuade an initially sceptical public of the need for change. As an example of societal reform it is particularly resonant now, when the bar for public tolerance of interventionist public health measures has perhaps been reset to a higher level with the extraordinary global government-led response to coronavirus. In the coming months, many ministers and mayors will look to the handful of countries which have managed to transform their national public health outcomes to see how it was done. If they use Finland as an example, a vital part of the story is where it all began.

The war on cholesterol

I am approaching the end of my very long chat with Pukka Peska, the Finnish doctor who is one of the true pioneers of modern public health, when a question occurs: how many early deaths does he think the programme he devised and led has saved? Peska says that he and some colleagues had once sat down to calculate this. They eventually worked out that if mortality rates had stayed the same as they were when he began his work in the early 1970s, over the next thirty years alone there would have been an additional 250,000 deaths among people aged under seventy-five. This is not, it should be added, a calculation taking in all of Finland, just one region of it, and not an especially populous one at that. It is, I tell him with some understatement, not bad going for a career achievement. Peska laughs. 'This is public health,' he says. 'Of course, when I became involved, I believed that we could have results, but never, ever could I believe that the chronic disease epidemic would change so dramatically.'[5]

There is an important point to make here. The disease epidemic Peska was trying to curb was the same foe as faced by Dr Jerry Morris: cardiovascular disease, and in particular fatal heart attacks. But Peska was not, at least initially, seeking to change the health odds via physical activity. His first targets were diet and tobacco. However, as an example of turning a population away from habits which were killing them young, Peska's work has enormous relevance for modern efforts to promote movement. Amid the admittedly specialist world of public health programmes tackling the diseases of lifestyle, his example is perhaps the most celebrated and influential of all.

It took place in North Karelia, the fairly remote Finnish region of which Joensuu is the capital, which at the start of the 1970s was among the poorest parts of the country, heavily reliant on agriculture and forestry. At the time, North Karelia had the highest coronary mortality rate in Finland, which in turn had the worst such record in the world. An enormously high proportion of those who died were men, often in middle age. Something had to be done, Finnish officials decided. In late 1971, they formed a committee tasked with finding ways to turn this around. The main investigator, sent to the region with a mandate to save lives, was Peska.

'I became involved as a very young doctor,' he recalls. 'At that time it was a crazy, crazy idea. In North Karelia, our problem at that time was not obesity or physical inactivity, because people were farmers and lumberjacks – physically very active. But the diet was absolutely crazy. Enormous amounts of animal fat and dairy fat, practically no vegetables, no fruit, and also enormous amounts of smoking. Those were our problems. But the principles are still the same: how to influence human behaviours, in individuals or in population-wide behaviour.'

The years of work led by Peska and his team essentially wrote the modern guidebook for how to transform public health. At one level, there was – after some persuasion – significant political help, with Finland passing early legislation to restrict smoking, including a ban on all tobacco advertising in 1976. The other element was a huge programme of public information material, and endless other ways to cajole, persuade or otherwise urge people – mainly the men, in this case – in North Karelia to stop smoking and change their diets.

From just 1972 to 1977, Peska's team pumped out material for 1,500 newspaper articles, about one a day, and distributed almost 100,000 Father's Day cards carrying healthy messages. On smoking, they ran 'quit and win' contests. They arranged a cholesterol-lowering competition between two villages, only for forty villages to decide they wanted to take part. The winning community saw average adult cholesterol levels fall by 11 per cent in just two months. At the same time, local authorities tried to help farmers move away from the dairy-based agriculture dominant in the region, providing support for them to grow berries instead.

By any imaginable metric, the long-term results were stunning. In slightly over three decades the annual age-adjusted cardiac death rate among men aged thirty-five to sixty-four, the main target for the work, dropped by 85 per cent in North Karelia. Death rates for many cancers, not least for ones related to smoking, also fell significantly, as did overall mortality rates for both genders. Other figures were equally impressive. The male smoking rate fell from 52 per cent to 31 per cent. The proportion of people who routinely spread butter on their bread went from more than 80 per cent to below 10 per cent, while the numbers of men who ate vegetables virtually every day increased four-fold.[6]

Peska is impatient with the idea that the success was in some way a result of a distinctive Finnish culture in which people are particularly receptive to official advice. 'When I speak about this in other countries, very often the comments are, "Oh, that's easy for you because the Finns are such nice people; it won't work for us",' he tells me. 'But the obstacles were enormous in the '70s. Changing human behaviour is difficult everywhere. And there's no magic bullet. This was all new. When we said we wanted to do community-based prevention with heart disease, the cardiologists said, "What the hell are you talking about? Community-based prevention? We don't even know how to prevent it among individuals." But the thing is that if you want to change behaviours, it has to be changed in society, with the physical and social environment, and I think that's critical also for physical activity.'

Peska says that during the 1990s, as researchers started to see more overweight people, they realised that with patterns of work changing, physical inactivity was becoming a new problem. And despite the immeasurably more healthy diet, BMI levels rose over the period of the project.

He snorts when I mention the 'nanny state' objection raised by British politicians over such lifestyle-based policies. 'It's a terrible statement,' he fumes. 'You can still behave as you want. But you just have the support to have a healthy lifestyle. Most smokers would like to stop. Most overweight people would like to lose weight. So it is giving support to people to do things that they want. And when you speak about the nanny state, we must also remember children. I don't think they should have free choice. I think it is the role of schools and society to guide children.'

In terms of lessons for other countries, the North Karelia project particularly highlights two elements. One is the vital importance of community buy-in, making sure people know why it is a good idea for the project to succeed. For example, Peska's team worked closely with housewives' associations, given at the time it was almost always the women of a household who bought and prepared all the food. Reaching the housewives was also important because while the men saw smoking as a rare pleasure in a generally deprived area, it was the families who experienced the aftermath of so many early male deaths.

A 1990s report into the project, co-written by Peska, reprints a series of heart-rending letters sent to the public health team from bereaved local women, with one describing heart disease as 'our family curse'. Another wrote to tell the researchers that her husband had died of a heart attack: 'He had one five years ago, followed by two more; the third one took him. He was a heavy smoker, which certainly contributed to it and damaged his heart. I hope that this project can bring understanding and help to many, so that people do not have to lose their health at their best age.'[7]

The other lesson is the need for complete political support. Peska, who went on to become a politician himself for a period, among many other later roles, says this took time. 'Gradually, when things started to move, politicians became more interested,' he says. 'We got the tobacco legislation very early, some rules about food production. So policy is important. But how do you move politicians? That comes back to the media. I've been a member of parliament twice, and rational arguments are obviously important, but what really moves politicians is when they see that voters are moving. The voter is the king.'

Some Finns do understandably grumble about what can be the country's arguably sanitised international reputation as a paradise of universally excellent education and equality, presided over by a caring government which promotes public health. They point to serious social problems, not to mention significant political divisions illustrated by the rise of the True Finns, the populist right-wing, anti-immigrant party who are now the second-biggest force in parliament, if nonetheless shut out of the coalition in which Krista Kiuru serves.

But almost fifty years on from the start of Pukka Peska's work, it seems clear that the politicians have listened to him. Kiuru tells me the North Karelia project was seen as 'a challenge' to the rest of the country, and that the political consensus has very much been changed. Even the True Finns support the interventionist approach to public health, she says.

There is similar near-unanimity over other policies, such as the €500 million spent every year on providing free, nutritious meals to every schoolchild, which was Kiuru's responsibility in a former role as education minister. She recalls how one MP objected to the cost. She responded by taking him to eat one of the meals. Seeing how healthy and tasty it was, he changed his mind. 'This is something which is carrying Finland towards the future,' she says. 'It will save us money in the long term. It is investing in people, investing in kids. Finns are basically quite motivated taxpayers – if they can see that there is a greater good which will come from it.'

The mention of tax is important. If Finland's example tells us anything, it is that the big changes need the sort of resources that can only really come from central government. In 1980, Finland passed what was known as the Sports Act, giving significant central funding for new sports facilities and creating local officials to oversee the process. A central registry of sports sites now lists about 30,000 venues – one for every 175 or so Finns. An updated Sports Act in 1999 expanded the scope to more everyday physical activity, providing money for cycle routes and small local parks.[8]

A lot of the efforts around activity are focused on young people – it is no coincidence that the Winter Cycling Congress opened at a primary school. In the last chapter we heard about Finnish Schools on the Move, a government programme to increase movement among young people, for example with active lessons, or the option for pupils to stand as they learn.

In Joensuu, I meet Joonas Niemi, one of the lead coordinators from Finnish Schools on the Move, who is there to discuss promoting active school travel. Year-round across Finland about 65 per cent of children walk or cycle to school, a figure which rises to 80 per cent outside winter.[9] He is talking at the Winter Cycling Congress about a project in which his team lent cameras to students to film their bike rides to and from school, so they could point out places on the route they found worrying or unsafe. Inside schools, the goal is to add an hour of physical activity to every school day, including movement in lessons.[10]

A strand of Finnish Schools on the Move, known as Joy in Motion, sends teams into kindergartens to help teachers promote activity. Nina Korhonen, a former kindergarten teacher who leads the project in the education ministry, says it is as much about changing attitudes as anything else. 'It doesn't really cost much,' she tells. 'How much does it cost to have children running around? It doesn't need anything big. You just need to get the teachers to change their approach. When I was trained as a teacher we were taught to keep the children quiet. We tell them it's good for the kids to run around.'[11]

Sanna Ojajärvi is yet another public employee who is paid to get young people moving. Her work with the Network of Finnish Cycling Municipalities, a cross-council group promoting active travel, involves spreading the bike message in schools and kindergartens, including children as young as three. With younger children, she says, the best promotion is games, such as one where she blows bubbles and they have to cycle through and catch them. 'What the teachers are afraid of is the kids just messing around,' Ojajärvi says. 'But usually nobody falls. And if a small kid falls off it's perfectly normal – if you learn how to cycle, of course you'll fall off. But it's not dangerous.'[12]

Trying to reset childhood

Finland is not the only country trying to push the pro-movement message for children. Chris Wright is head of wellbeing at the UK's Youth Sports Trust, and he is as passionate about the subject as any Finn. His organisation runs programmes in nurseries and kindergartens in economically deprived areas of England, promoting movement-based learning, also trying to persuade parents to let their toddlers run around elsewhere. This is hugely important work. If you remember the statistic from Chapter 1, only 9 per cent of British children under five currently meet the age-group recommendation that, once they can walk, they should amass at least three hours of physical activity a day.[13]

I had been due to see one of these projects in action at a nursery in Minehead, a coastal town in Somerset, in southwest England. However, the coronavirus lockdown put a stop to this. Wright tells me the area around Minehead has been shown to have England's lowest levels of social mobility. It is thus a focus for the activity programme, given that movement in the early years of a child's life has been shown to be key to not just their physical development, but progress in a series of other areas.

'Movement and play in the early years can help to develop literacy, language communication, building relationships, and being more confident individuals,' Wright tells me. 'The attributes that children get from playing and moving have a direct correlation then on being able to read, being able to grip a pen, being able to sit down and concentrate on tasks. It's fundamental to children's development. If they're not moving, then, you know, the evidence will tell you that they're not developing.'[14]

Two years of work in nurseries like the one in Minehead have shown 'a demonstrable difference not just on children's activity levels, but their language, their ability to form positive relationships and their confidence in their learning and also in who they are', Wright tells me.

He is critical of the English school curriculum's apparent lack of interest in physical development, saying that even in kindergarten settings it can be 'quite narrow' and insufficiently play-based. This, he argues, has to change: 'It's adults that stop children from moving, and what we're trying to do is unlock their ability to be able to move, and reset childhood to a certain degree. If these weeks with COVID-19 have taught us anything, it's that movement is probably more important now than it ever has been. You can have an education system that, of course, educates children to be able to pursue the careers and the life that they want, but they also need the fundamentals of wellbeing in order to be able to achieve that. I think that's the message that's slowly starting to creep across the system.'

Talking to Wright is inspirational. But there is one glaring difference between his efforts, however persuasive and effective, and the work done by people like Nina Korhonen and Joonas Niemi. They are civil servants, part of a system of government specifically geared towards creating activity in everyday life. In contrast, the Youth Sports Trust is a charity. By the standards of many charities it is relatively well funded, with an overall income last year of £11.6 million, a mixture of government grants and sponsorship. But in national terms, even for just one aspect of public health, such a sum is virtually an irrelevance. It amounts to just under 0.02 per cent of the budget of the Department for Education,[15] against whose more instinctively anti-movement approach the charity often campaigns. If ministers gave Wright an official post with a bigger budget, sufficient political backing and enough time, I'm sure he could transform the physical future for the UK's children. But at the moment it's just not a fair fight.

It is a contrast you see again and again when you examine the approach to tackling inactivity in places like the UK, as against centrally led programmes as seen in Finland, or even with the decades of consistent spending on and support for cycle infrastructure in the Netherlands and Denmark. There are British success stories, but as with the exemplary work of Chris Wright, and the Daily Mile, which we saw in the preceding chapter, they are invariably private or charitable enterprises, reliant on occasional official help or, as with the Daily Mile, the largesse of a multinational company as sponsor.

Another notable example of this is Parkrun, the weekly 5km mass run which since starting in 2004 has spread both across the UK and to dozens of other countries, and now claims 3 million participants worldwide. Parkrun is fascinating in that it is an ostensibly sports-based event – a timed run over a set distance – which has nonetheless developed a culture which makes it welcoming to participants ranging from elite athletes to previously inactive first-timers, as well as those who simply volunteer.

Parkrun started life as the Bushy Park Time Trial, set up by keen runner Paul Sinton-Hewitt as primarily a social event, since at the time he was injured and had depression. From a single venue in southwest London and a first outing involving thirteen runners and three volunteers, it has expanded into a near-ubiquitous feature of parks on a Saturday morning, run by an associated charity which is heavily involved in wider physical activity efforts.

Chrissie Wellington, Parkrun's head of wellbeing, says that despite the name, it is less a race than what she calls 'a community-led social event centred on activity'. She explains: 'What is central is that Parkrun can be anything you want it to be. And that's really, really important. People consume Parkrun in many different ways. Some just come along for the post-event coffee; others see it very much as a time trial and are using it either as a target event or as a means to achieve a target time in a race. So the timed element is an important part of Parkrun. And competitiveness with oneself or with others can be important. But it is not the central kind of *raison d'être* of Parkrun, as it might be for other physical activity.'[16]

You cannot simply turn up to a Parkrun. Participants, whether running or volunteering, must register on a website and bring a printed barcode, which is scanned each time they take part. This creates a huge database of who takes part and how often, and how fast they go if they run. Because the registration form includes a question on current activity levels, this also tracks those who change their lifestyles. Part of Wellington's role is to use these statistics to try to make Parkrun better at reaching more people, as well as having to deal with the fifty-plus annual requests from academics and universities wanting to use Parkrun's database for research projects.

There are now around 6 million people signed up, even if

more than half never make it to an event. The data, Wellington says, shows the event is attracting lots of people who are 'starting out on their journey to being active', with up to 7 per cent saying they are totally immobile when they register. 'Evidence suggests those that are less active are not only increasing their activity through Parkrun but are increasing their activity outside of it,' Wellington says.

The benefits are even seen in volunteers, whose duties often involve them walking greater distances than they would usually, and who then can end up being more active in other aspects of their lives. There is evidence, Wellington says, that the volunteers see the biggest life changes of anyone: 'It really does show us that involvement in Parkruns isn't simply beneficial due to walking or running at the event, and that volunteering is as important, if not more.'

Again, it is hard to overstate the value of the work Parkrun manages to achieve. But once more, this has to be seen in context. It is an even smaller charity than the Youth Sports Trust, with an annual income of just over £4 million and a heavy reliance on volunteering and goodwill. Like the Daily Mile, it operates in the slightly precarious intersection between campaigning and an almost official role. In the case of Parkrun, this includes links with doctors' surgeries, so GPs can 'prescribe' taking part in Parkruns to patients who arrive with conditions associated with inactivity. So far it has connected to around 1,500 GP practices, almost a fifth of all those in the UK. It also helps arrange Parkruns in more than twenty prisons and young offenders' institutions, something as much connected to welfare and rehabilitation as fitness.

All this is admirable and does a huge amount of good, but it remains fundamentally different to the more centrally planned approach adopted by other governments, where activity can be added into every aspect of official policy. To take yet another example from Finland, when I see Nina Korhonen to discuss her work in making kindergartens more active, we decide to meet at Helsinki's very new and hugely grand central library, a light-filled modern space with two excellent cafés, one of which we sit in. In keeping with the more communal Finnish approach, like many of the country's libraries it does much more than just lend books and serve very good coffee. There are meeting rooms and recording studios which can be booked for free, as well as sewing machines and even a 3D printer. You can also borrow sports equipment, while some other libraries can lend a pedal-powered cargo bike able to carry heavy loads.

This is not to say that this is the only model for every country. Helsinki's library cost nearly €100 million, and it takes a certain political consensus for voters to accept the levels of tax needed to fund not just projects like this, but the wages of Joonas Niemi's Finnish Schools on the Move teams, as well as one sports facility per 175 people.

But the experience of physical activity programmes across the world all point in the same direction: for all the amazing work of people like Chrissie Wellington and Chris Wright, if you want true, population-wide benefits, relying on charities is not enough. This is the work of governments.

Winning the obesity battle

None of this is to say that Finland now has the problem of inactivity solved. It remains very much an ongoing process, particularly when it comes to young people. The mammoth and ongoing Global Report Card study on childhood activity levels across forty-nine countries, mentioned in Chapter 1, gives Finland an 'A' score for efforts in schools, but notes that even with this only around a third of its nine- to fifteen-year-olds manage the recommended hour a day of sufficient exertion. This is much better than the UK, even if different reporting methods mean there is not a direct comparison. For the UK, only about 20 per cent for the broad group aged five to fifteen meet the activity minimums, a figure which is inflated by the generally higher activity levels among younger children.[17]

But, as also mentioned in the first chapter, when it comes to childhood activity, one country shines through: Slovenia. The tiny former Yugoslav state, which became formally independent only in 1991, is becoming known as the new activity success story in town, and one which has seen this achieved within a generation.

So rapid has been the progress that you can see it, starkly, in national statistics. Slovenia's figures for adult activity are, to be blunt, fairly underwhelming. These are broadly the same as for the UK, with about 60 per cent of people reaching recommended weekly exertion levels,[18] even if more precise comparison is tricky as, again, the two countries release figures for different age points. In contrast, the Global Report Card study gives Slovenia by far the most glowing write-up of the forty-nine countries surveyed for activity levels in children, noting that more than 80 per cent of those aged six to nineteen are reported as meeting the one-hour-a-day threshold for activity.[19]

I go to Ljubljana to try to find out how this happened. The Slovenian capital is very much a city of two parts, with the beautiful and tranquil old town surrounded by a bigger and considerably less lovely mass of busy roads and 1960s-vintage offices and apartment blocks. When it comes to everyday activity, the city is, similarly, something of a mixed bag. There are numerous cycle lanes, with about 10 per cent of all trips made by bike. I spend my day successfully and safely navigating between various interviews on one of Ljubljana's public bikes. But simultaneously, the moment you move outside the mainly pedestrianised old town, the roads are often wide and generally jammed with gridlocked cars.

Polona Demšar Mitrovič, who is head of sustainable mobility at the Ministry of Infrastructure, based inside one of the many 1960s office blocks, tells me that outside the capital, Slovenia is even more dominated by motor vehicles, in part because of the terrible state of public transport, with no city metro systems, a single-track intercity rail network and 'awful' cross-country buses. 'When I came to work for this ministry ten years ago, it was still called the Ministry for Roads,' she says. 'It was all about building roads and highways. When we started this programme, my colleagues called me "the green one" – meaning the crazy one.'[20]

Demšar Mitrovič's role is to push cycling and public transport. Enjoyably blunt about her ministerial bosses, she says that most of the support in this area, both financially and politically, has come from the EU rather than Slovenian politicians, who she describes as being stuck in the past. 'They just want to build more and more road space,' she says. 'They don't realise that it's about using the existing roads in a better way. In the same EU funding document where we were seeking money for sustainable travel, we also asked for money to pay for an extra lane on the Ljubljana ring road. It's a strange situation – we want a third lane, to bring more traffic into the city, but at the same time we want to close streets in the city to cars.'

Other areas of activity promotion have proved more fruitful. About twenty minutes' cycle ride away, in another looming office block, Mojca Gobec, head of public health in the Ministry of Health, says she has seen at least some politicians starting to listen. Her department leads a huge, ten-year nationwide campaign based on greater activity and better diets, called *Dober Tek*, a pun using the Slovenian pre-meal equivalent of *bon appetit*, which also has a literal translation connected to movement.

'Our tourist strategy is based on Slovenia being an active, healthy and green destination,' Gobec says. 'If we're offering that, it should be natural that we're trying to live that kind of life. We've come quite a long way because the Ministry of Sport used to see elite athletes as a priority, the Olympics and so on. But now it's more and more about everyday physical activities.'[21]

As mentioned, by far the greatest success in Slovenia's physical activity record has come with children. Like Finland, this is the result of many years of government-led intervention, even if the feel is somewhat different. If Finland's approach is a typically Nordic, social democrat–type, Slovenia's programme for young people and schools feels almost communist – and, in fact, did originate in Yugoslav times.

Since 1982, in April every single student at all of Slovenia's primary and secondary schools has undergone the same battery of standardised tests and measurements: height, weight and skinfold body fat, then eight physical tests, including a standing jump, 600m run, 60m run, and a bent arm hang. The participation rate is virtually universal, higher even than that for compulsory childhood vaccinations, with results added to a database now covering more than half the country's population. Children are ranked against national percentile scores, meaning modern children can compare their rankings against children from the 1980s, in some cases including their own parents.

Gregor Starc, an exercise scientist at the University of Ljubljana, who co-runs the programme, known as Slofit, says the results alone can prompt action: 'Some parents are shocked when they realise their kids are not doing as well as them, so realise they need to change,' he says. 'Some families have altered their entire lifestyles.' But the main focus is on activity in schools, something Starc says was a deliberate policy choice: 'We saw that whenever countries were counting on parents to take care of the physical fitness and physical activity of children, it failed. That's why we focused on schools. So now Slovenia has one of the highest qualities of physical education teaching in the world, and the infrastructure is excellent.'[22]

As mentioned in the last chapter, every Slovenian school has two gyms and an outdoor play area, as well as track and field facilities. Beyond PE lessons in the curriculum, each child has five 'sports days' per year, and is given another week off for outdoor activities, often held at former Yugoslav army bases now run by the education ministry. 'All the equipment is there, the bicycles, the bows and arrows, the skis, climbing equipment, whatever they want,' Starc says.

Such has been the success of all this that Slovenia identifies itself as the only country in the world where child obesity rates are going down. 'There are other countries that have a levelling off of obesity, but in our country, it has gone down from 2010/11. The rates are going down and physical fitness is going up,' Starc says. Fitness has particularly improved in girls, he explains, in part due to wider social changes: 'When I was a child, we were playing cowboys and Indians outside, the girls would only be nurses, tending to the wounded. But nowadays, they do everything – play football, they play whatever they want to. Girls today are 20 per cent fitter than their mothers were. The boys are close to fathers, but still like a percent below. But they're getting there. If we don't do anything stupid in terms of politics, they will catch up within five years.'

This is not to say that everything is well. A particular worry is the small minority of children who are morbidly obese, the proportion of which is not falling. This is, Starc says, a wider problem: 'We cannot repair them in school. They need a holistic approach, and probably the entire family has to be involved.'

This is perhaps an obvious point, but also one worth stressing: for all the importance of the state in leading national health efforts, official action cannot do everything. Slovenia can provide the best sports facilities possible in schools, and spend thirty years monitoring fitness, but no child can be properly active without at least some family support. It was the same for Puska Pekka. Even after his team pulled every lever of officialdom and government to improve public health, the key to change was persuading housewives in North Karelia that they could make changes in their own households to stop their menfolk getting heart attacks.

At the same time, it is notable that the two countries in Europe most associated with recent improvements in activity levels both take a notably interventionist position. This will not, and cannot, solve everything. But for all the valiant and inspiring efforts of people like Chris Wright and Chrissie Wellington, and the very real benefits they bring to thousands of people, it is inevitable that charities and voluntary groups, however much they seek to integrate into official public health programmes, can never have the same reach. It's just not realistic.

Does this mean countries like the UK are condemned to limp on with an ever-growing personal and societal burden connected to immobile living? For all Pukka Peska might dismiss the idea of the Finns being special, can other countries change? The answer for now is that we don't know. But one thing is clear: other countries have shown they are able to act decisively. A lesson from the coronavirus pandemic has been that when it comes to governments interfering directly in the lives of their populations to keep them healthy, things can change very quickly indeed.

Next steps:

If a lot of countries, like the UK, are not as motion-friendly as Finland or Slovenia, that can in part be because MPs and councillors don't really consider it an issue. Many politicians have told me that car drivers tend to be much more vocal than people who more commonly travel by bike or on foot. So if you want a more human-friendly local area, it can be worth making that known.

10

So What Now? A New Era of Health

I can remember exactly where I was at the moment the British prime minister, Boris Johnson, announced that the country was going into enforced lockdown to try to slow the spread of coronavirus. As with so many key political moments over the past few years – and perhaps not the best image for the message of this book – I was sitting hunched over a laptop, typing up facts and quotes to turn them into a news story as fast as possible.

People were ordered to stay at home in all circumstances other than for vital work, purchasing necessities, for medical needs, or one form of exercise. They would be fined if they did not, under a law rushed through parliament earlier that day, carried with no dissenting voices, and without even a formal vote among MPs. The restrictions were onerous and unprecedented, even in wartime. They would jeopardise millions of jobs and send the national economy into a nosedive. And yet the public were hugely in favour. Many, in fact, had wanted the rules imposed weeks earlier. All this, of course, was being done under the justification of saving lives. Similar regulations were imposed in many dozens of other countries, most likely sparing hundreds of thousands, if not millions, of people who would otherwise have died from the virus.

I've mentioned several times in the preceding chapters that this book is being written amid this lockdown. In fact the process has more or less completely coincided with the peak of restrictions in the UK. And it is an undeniable paradox to have spent my days chronicling successive government failures over one public health disaster when, at precisely the same moment, many of them are tackling another life-threatening crisis with genuine boldness.

In terms of scale, inactivity is not quite so acute as coronavirus, which, according to the scientific modelling which eventually persuaded Johnson to confine people to their homes, could have killed between 250,000 and 500,000 people in the UK alone if nothing was done.[1] Coronavirus has also provoked a particularly urgent response by being new, rapid in its destructiveness, and directly fatal. In contrast, someone in their twenties who flops down on a sofa tonight might not start to feel the impact of an inactive lifestyle for several decades, and then only through the impact of various chronic illnesses.

All that said, it must be remembered that inactivity is by no means the only public health emergency treated with at least some neglect by many governments. Air pollution, much of it from motor vehicles, is responsible for anything up to around 40,000 deaths a year in the UK,[2] and yet ministers have fought court cases to avoid being held even to minimum EU standards over clean air.[3] Similarly, while road casualties have fallen greatly over the decades, if it was terrorism which still killed an average of five people a day and left another hundred in hospital, many with injuries that will permanently transform their lives, you can bet that this toll would not be normalised and largely ignored.

This dual approach to the health of nations puzzled me long before COVID. But it seems all the more relevant now. If governments can treat a virus as a national emergency, why can't more of them deal with the many, well-proved repercussions of population-wide inactivity with at least the same seriousness and focus as the Finns or Slovenians? I decided to take advantage of my job and ask a few politicians.

I spoke to Jeremy Hunt after coronavirus had arrived in the UK, but a couple of weeks ahead of the lockdown. The Conservative MP spent just under six years as Health Secretary, the longest period anyone has held the job in Britain. After coming second to Johnson in the race to succeed Theresa May as prime minister, he now chairs the committee of backbench MPs who examine health issues. Hunt is fascinating in that he almost epitomises the approach to inactivity I have seen so often from British politicians: a clearly sincere personal commitment to, and understanding of, the issues, but one which either becomes a bit elusive when it comes to actual policies, or finds itself frustrated by a wall of official inertia.

Hunt is effusive about his own activity regime, saying one of the benefits of losing a ministerial post was being able to cycle freely around London again. His last job in government had been as Foreign Secretary, a role that comes with 24-hour police protection. While the police officers would happily cycle with him if asked, Hunt tells me, it was complex to arrange and, as he puts it, 'I never got my cycling act in order.'

He describes himself as a 'passionate believer' in everyday physical activity and is a fan of the Daily Mile programme. Hunt, who has young children, is particularly keen on more movement in schools. 'When I was Health Secretary I asked the chief medical officer whether she would be willing to give public advice to all schools that every child should have an hour of exercise a day,' Hunt tells me. 'I was really shocked when my own children became old enough and they went to a state school, they weren't getting an hour of exercise automatically built into their daily routine.'

However, in an experience echoing that of Elaine Wyllie with the Daily Mile, it was not that straightforward. And remember, rather than an individual headteacher, like Wyllie, seeking change, this was one of the most powerful politicians in the land. 'It was a real battle with the Department for Education, because their view is that schools are overloaded with instructions and requirements, and we were starting to undermine the autonomy of heads because we've overloaded the curriculum,' Hunt recalls.

On more general efforts to push activity, Hunt argues that the key in the UK is to not be too prescriptive: 'I think the way that it works is that in a free country, you have to take public opinion with you. And the trick as a government is to be a little bit ahead of public opinion on issues like this, guiding public opinion. But not so far ahead that you put everyone off and you lose them.' To an extent, this is the 'voter is king' maxim expressed by Pukka Peska in the last chapter. But what perhaps differentiates someone like Hunt from a Finnish politician, apart of course from several fewer decades of national focus on public health ideas, is a greater sense of caution when it comes to nudging, or leading, voters onwards. Hunt says: 'Public health campaigns always have to deal with the complaint of being nanny state. And so there is always a sensitivity, there's always a constituency dead against any kind of nanny state interventions.'[4]

There it is: the phrase so disliked by Peska – the fear of a government being seen as too interfering in telling individuals how to protect their welfare. And yet, when I speak to Hunt, his own party is weeks away from openly ordering an entire nation what to do to avert a health crisis. You could argue that coronavirus is different in that the threat can be transmitted, so it is a matter of communal rather than individual responsibility. However, as we've seen across this book, personal choice also tends to be a moot concept when it comes to physical activity. Being unable to cycle to work because of speeding motor traffic is not the same as absorbing viral droplets from another passenger coughing on a packed train. But both are firmly outside the individual's control.

To get another perspective, I talk to Sarah Wollaston, a family doctor who became a Conservative MP, before then defecting to the Liberal Democrats. Now out of parliament, when we speak she has just finalised re-joining the medical register to help with coronavirus efforts. As an MP Wollaston chaired the health committee now led by Hunt, which under her leadership produced a report into the inactivity crisis, which called for considerably more official action on the issue.

Wollaston's opinion is that none of the health ministers she tackled on the issue, Hunt included, seemed to really get it. 'It's just lip service,' she tells me. 'They say they take it seriously. But it's one thing to say, "Yes, yes, we know all this is terribly important," but it's another thing to put in place the policy that makes it a reality. It doesn't just happen by telling people to go out and exercise more. Promotion is all very well, but as with any public health programme, it's people who are already active and well informed who pick up on the advice, and you just end up with widening health inequalities.'

This is particularly the case, she says, over walking and cycling: 'The power is all in the car lobby. It's not with the cycling lobby. Until we shift that and you have ministers prepared to be bold and to ring-fence a sufficient amount of the transport budget to active travel, it's never going to happen.'[5]

For a final point of view I seek out someone who has dealt with the subject in two ways. Andy Burnham was, like Hunt, the Health Secretary, holding the role in the Labour government of Gordon Brown. He is now mayor of Greater Manchester, where he employs Chris Boardman to transform the city for cyclists and walkers, as we saw in Chapter 5. Burnham has a perhaps more Finnish opinion on the nanny state. 'You know the quote about the nanny state, don't you?' he tells me mischievously. 'People who complain about the nanny state are usually people who had nannies when they were children.'

Burnham argues that one of the difficulties in central government pushing cohesively for more physical activity is that it is, as he puts it, 'an orphan policy', which falls between the remits of several departments. 'It's not quite the Department for Culture, Media and Sport, because they're more sport,' he explains. 'With Communities and Local Government, it's not really top of their list. And with Health, they think of hospitals before they think of parks and active living. So it kind of falls between the cracks, and therefore it's never been properly championed from a national perspective. And yet, it is the answer to so many things, and not just health.'

Could this change with coronavirus? Burnham believes it might, not least because of the need to transform the way people move around cities, with continued social distancing meaning a drastic reduction in public transport capacity. A couple of days before speaking to me, Burnham had been on a conference call with Johnson and the mayors of other English cities, including London, to discuss ways to prevent gridlock if many thousands of extra people try to drive to work. Burnham recounts what the prime minister told them: 'We were given what sounded like very active instructions to prioritise cycling and walking infrastructure.'[6]

This opens up the possibility of a tipping point for activity, not just in the UK but in numerous other places. It could arguably be seen as an accidental victory, almost a by-product, given that the main impetus in reshaping urban transport priorities would be to avoid crowds on trains and buses, and then in turn to prevent roads seizing up from a rush to car travel. To an extent, this is immaterial: just as your body doesn't care whether its activity comes through formal exercise or routine exertion, the health benefits from more people using new bike lanes or widened pavements are exactly the same, no matter why they were constructed.

That said, there are other public health issues at play, and signs that some in government are aware of them. As mentioned earlier, a series of initial studies have noted the way coronavirus appears particularly deadly not just in older people but in those who are obese or have conditions such as high blood pressure, type 2 diabetes and cardiovascular disease, all of which are closely linked to inactivity. But one research paper from a US professor of exercise science, David Nieman, so recent that it was published only six days before I type these words, makes a more explicit link between the two areas. Coronavirus, Nieman argues, is 'a wake-up call' over the globe's increasingly poor long-term health. All similar viruses, he notes, have notably higher mortality rates in people who are physically inactive, meaning the promotion of movement should be among the 'primary prevention strategies against respiratory illnesses'.[7] Has this message resonated? It's hard to tell, and, at least in the UK, you could imagine some politicians viewing it as a move into nanny state territory. But certainly some people I have talked to inside Downing Street appear to understand the point.

The other side of the equation is whether people, having been through the coronavirus restrictions, will become more accepting of subsequent interventionist government policies, particularly if they might improve outcomes in future outbreaks. Burnham, for one, thinks this is possible: 'There is such an opportunity here, and I did sort of hear in Boris Johnson's voice that he might get that. Time will tell. But it's an opportunity I don't think we'll ever get again in quite this form. There is a public appetite to not go back to business as usual – people want this to be a moment of positive change, in many ways.'

Burnham says he has been thinking about the political transformation after voters removed Winston Churchill from office in 1945, despite him leading the nation through the war, with the Labour government bequeathing the UK its National Health Service and social security system. 'I feel like I understand that a bit more now, with coronavirus,' Burnham explains. 'You look at the world through a new lens when you have a moment like this. I think the public do have a more public-spirited sentiment.'

The double narrative

The parallel with the post-war period is one several people are making. A few days after talking to Burnham I speak to a former colleague of his, Ed Miliband, not officially in connection with this book, but for my day job. Miliband, the ex-Labour leader, is now responsible for industrial policy with the party, and is explaining his hopes that economic recovery efforts after the coronavirus lockdown will be centred on green issues, which would include more active travel.

'It's a contemporary equivalent of what happened after 1945,' Miliband tells me. 'It's never too early to start thinking about the future, to think about what kind of world we want to build as we emerge from this crisis. I do think that there's a public mood about this. I think we owe it to have a sort of reassessment of what really matters in our society, and how do we build something better for the future.'[8]

On the same day I speak to Miliband, in fact at more or less the same time, a spokesman for Boris Johnson tells journalists, including one of my colleagues, that the prime minister is devising plans for a new approach to the nation's health in the wake of his own near-fatal encounter with coronavirus. He is, we are told, extremely serious about this.[9] No more than an hour after that, some other news emerges: my own city, London, is to close off large sections of the centre to all vehicles apart from buses, bicycles and pedestrians, at a stroke creating one of the biggest traffic-free areas in the world.[10] It's the kind of plan that even a few months earlier would have seemed an impossible dream, something that would need years of consultation. Now, the work is scheduled to be completed within six weeks.

This is suddenly moving from the unlikely into the downright strange. There are two narratives unfolding with this book. The first is the one I have outlined over the preceding chapters: a centuries-old story about the gradual eradication of everyday physical movement from so many lives, and a reluctance on the part of ministers and officials to engage properly with the repercussions. In parallel, and as I write those same chapters, the discourse on public health in the outside world is changing at an unprecedented pace. It is no longer just that governments are taking concerted action on the different public health crisis of coronavirus. Many of them are now responding to the challenge by introducing some of the most radical measures ever seen which could reintroduce large-scale physical activity.

It is thus the fate of this book to end on something of a cliffhanger, one where the reader will have the inevitable benefit of several more months of knowledge. It's impossible to tell where all this will go. It is entirely feasible that emergency cycle lanes and expanded pavements in Paris, Milan, New York, London, Manchester, Liverpool and countless other cities stay in place, bringing with them an upsurge in the number of people walking or cycling their way to the thirty minutes a day of health-enhancing activity, and beyond. Urban populations used to cleaner air could decide they don't want cars clogging their neighbourhoods again. The reborn, post-coronavirus economy and society could prompt a permanent, even if semi-accidental, shift towards more movement.

But it could all turn out very differently. In the coming weeks and months it might become clear that as people return to work but are banished from public transport, many decide they only feel safe driving. Spooked by gridlock, cities could instead remove bike lanes, make parking cheaper, express hopeful plat-itudes about an eventual shift towards electric cars as pollution levels soar again.

Right now, the former seems more likely, but the history of efforts to combat inactivity is littered with false dawns, for example the cycling boom that swept the US and several other countries following the 1973 oil price crisis, only to fizzle out. While I joke with friends and colleagues that the pace of change is now so rapid my book could end up being irrelevant before it is even published, the truth is that things are never so easy. As the Dutch and Danes showed, it takes decades to build an environment in which cycling becomes truly everyday and mainstream. And active travel is only one part of the picture. Jan Gehl has spent even longer trying to persuade people to reshape cities so human-scale movement becomes the norm, the obvious thing to do.

To extend the parallel made by others, like the Second World War, the coronavirus pandemic is so unutterably tragic and awful that it can feel anomalous to try to imagine benefits coming in its wake. But it is nonetheless vital to try to picture what might follow, and to hope it will be something better, something fairer. After decades of governments failing to take action over mass inactivity despite the overwhelming and direct evidence of the health crisis it creates, it would be curious if the eventual catalyst for change was something both different and unforeseen. But, as history has taught us again and again, when a revolution does arrive, it is not necessarily the one you were expecting.

The joy of tech

As you will have gathered by now, I've spent a long time thinking about physical activity, as well as talking to many people who think about it even more. And so, much as I have stressed several times that this is not a book of advice, it seems fair to use this final chapter to set out what I've learned along the way in these months as researcher, writer and occasional experimental subject/guinea pig.

One personal lesson is that despite an initial scepticism about the use of high-tech gadgets in monitoring and scrutinising activity levels, I in fact found they can be surprisingly useful to help you maintain a movement regime – or at least they can if you find the right device. Phone-based apps have played little part for me, mainly because I seemingly don't tend to carry my phone around with me enough to make them worthwhile. I downloaded Public Health England's Active Ten app, which has the excellent premise of trying to get people to record at least ten minutes of brisk walking a day. But, at least in lockdown, the app has recorded so little walking for me it is presumably just a matter of time before it remotely alerts my doctor, or sounds a noisy alarm.

Much more effective has been the wrist-worn fitness watch, with its built-in step counter and heart rate monitor. From a purely book-research point of view, the heart rate function was enormously useful in helping me work out how much activity I amassed during my usual, non-lockdown cycle commute, and at what intensity, as shown in Chapter 5. Such information, and particularly its ability to track bike rides and runs via GPS, veers significantly into the arena of exercise, and the watch is clearly aimed more at the recreational athlete than someone who just wants to build towards their 150 minutes a week of routine exertion, not least given it costs about £130. But for those, like Tom Watson, who prefer to observe their route to better health progress through charts and tables, this can still be very useful. The watch connects to a dedicated phone app, which over time amasses something of a personal health biography of heart rates, exertion levels and steps. It also tries to urge you into greater efforts by handing out slightly patronising virtual awards, for example a shiny, on-screen badge for reaching 15,000 steps in one day. Significantly more ludicrous was one portentously titled *I Am the Night*, which was awarded after I did nothing more notable than ride a bike after 10pm.

Most useful has been the watch's in-built step counter. As I detailed earlier in the book, as a target, 10,000 steps a day is largely arbitrary, and even clever, wrist-worn fitness devices are not always completely accurate. But they are a good general guide. There have been long days writing this book where I have looked up at 5pm to see I'd walked fewer than 2,000 steps, a very obvious reminder that I needed to do better the next day. The watch, a Garmin Forerunner 45, was lent to me by Wiggle, a UK-based online bike retailer who have an interest in active workplaces. Officially, it is mine to keep, but under UK journalism rules I can't accept gifts costing more than £50. My plan had been to give the device as a prize for my newspaper's annual charity auction. However, I might instead make a suitable donation myself and keep it. That's something of a testament to how habituated I have become to its daily stream of activity information, and how useful I now find this.

Sadly, the other item of technology I attached to myself for testing purposes was simultaneously the most enlightening and fascinating, but also the one device that people reading this book cannot just go out and buy for themselves. The tiny, thigh-attached plastic fob, weighing little more than a sheet of A4 paper, is very much a research-grade activity tracker, and while Sens, the Danish company who invented it, were able to indulge me with my one-off purchase, they don't usually take individual orders. In some ways this is a shame. If everyone was able to see a week of colour-coded movement charts showing how inactive they had been and how long they had sat down, it might shock at least a few into action.

The sensor's totals for how long I sit down every day, particularly at work, definitely provided the biggest personal wake-up call in writing this book. I was already generally aware I sat down excessively, and often without a break. But to see it translated into a daily total of nine or so hours, and to look at the chart with its long, afternoon sessions of continuous grey, had a real impact. I already sit less than I did, although the real test will happen when lockdown ends and I return to normal office life. I'm not quite at the stage of the inactivity professionals and their active applause, but I definitely get twitchy if I sit down for too long. That's some sort of progress.

Two other areas of activity research have been particularly eye-opening. One is the emphasis on strength or muscle training, which is so often neglected amid the focus on the 150 minutes a week of cardiovascular activity, and which I had certainly not thought much about. The other is reading so many research papers about the importance of at least some form of movement in helping process fats and sugars after a meal – a time when so many of us, me included, tend to slump on a sofa. In a newfound habit that very much strays from the mantra of everyday, integrated activity, but which I excuse as compensation for the long hours writing this book, in recent weeks I have found myself occasionally leaping up from in front of the TV to squat up and down while holding a barbell weight. It's definitely exercise. It's not especially elegant. But it is curiously satisfying.

If I were to try to convey some sort of more general lessons, I suppose the very condensed version would be to seek the more straightforward activity gains in whatever circumstances you face. So, if you have a garden and don't already tend it, that's guaranteed exertion. If you live in a flat, or work in an office block, take the stairs if you can. And if your job, like mine, involves sitting down, do whatever you can to get up more often.

But in terms of pure activity, the most effective way that most people can integrate and maintain more physicality in their lives is to walk around a bit more, or, if possible, use a bike. Walking has the advantage of being hugely straightforward, and flexible. So, for example, if you get a bus to work you can always get off a stop or two early some days. Even if you drive somewhere, seek out a distant corner of the car park, or a stopping point a few streets from your destination, picking up 1,000 or so steps every time. They all count, and they all add up, as do the health dividends.

It is when you're able to get about by bike, however, that the benefits really multiply. It's fair to say I am an unabashed advocate of everyday cycling for transport. I have written an entire book explaining why more of it is a good thing, not just for the rider but for everyone else. Particularly in places like the UK, it is not always easy, or in some cases even possible, to make cycling part of your regular transport regime. However, for those with shorter commutes, or other journeys, especially in urban areas, it can be more straightforward to do than many believe. If you are able to integrate cycling into your life, even if not every day, the benefits are almost too numerous to list, and go well beyond the remit of this book.

Aside even from the almost implausible health impacts, getting around by bike means you start to commune with your town or city in a different way, travelling at human-scale speed, but sufficiently rapid to cover significant distance. Streets and neighbourhoods suddenly open up. Rather than a destination being, say, three miles away, intangible and distant, it is suddenly twenty minutes' gentle ride, straightforward, predictable, punctual. Even the weather is more real. You feel the sting, or the caress, of the changing seasons against your face, noticing every alteration, every gradual shift. I wrote at the start of this book about how cycling helped unlock in me the sheer glee of feeling physically vital. This has never dimmed. There are times, even on the wearily familiar streets of my commute, when the realisation sweeps through me that I am privileged to use my body in this way, and that it won't be forever.

The one you'll keep doing

I am, however, not the expert here. For this book I talked to many of the world's leading researchers on activity, and how to better integrate it into our lives. At the end of our conversations, I would often ask how they found their own ways to remain physical. Several conceded that it took a certain amount of effort. But, as you can imagine, it was something they had all thought about a lot.

I-Min Lee, perhaps the modern academic world's most prominent activity researcher, grew up in Malaysia. There, she says, exercise was not particularly encouraged, and she only became active as a student of Ralph Paffenbarger, 'because it would be incredibly embarrassing not to exercise when you were doing physical activity research'. Very much identifying herself as someone who doesn't particularly enjoy formal exercise, Lee says she tries to walk or take stairs where she can, and has faced many of the same modern-world staircase pitfalls as me. 'In a lot of buildings I worry about going up the stairs, because I'm worried I'll be locked in the stairwell,' she tells me. 'Sometimes if I'm in a hotel, I'll get someone with me and I'll say, "Stay the other side, if I can't get back in, let me in." You don't want to be stuck in there in the middle of the night and having to open an alarmed door.'[11]

A lot of the researchers I talked to discussed how they try to stay active amid what are, in the main, sedentary jobs. As well as having a standing desk, Genevieve Healy tries to walk around her office as much as possible. 'It can be as straightforward as, instead of sending someone an email, you just go and have a brief standing meeting with them,' she says. William Haskell, for several decades one of the most influential people in the inactivity world, says that when he is at his office he will always 'stand up and go walk down the halls and talk to people rather than calling them on my phone'.[12]

On the day I speak to him, Richard Mackenzie had made being active part of his journey from the commuter town north of London where he lives, to his university – after dropping his infant son at nursery, he ran to the local train station, and then once in London ran to his workplace. This does, he admits, take a fair bit of planning and commitment: 'I would think that many other people would not do that. It's partly because of my job.' Mackenzie was in the army reserves, and says he formerly believed that activity 'had to be an hour of intense exercise, or I'm not doing anything worthwhile'. His mantra is now more forgiving: 'I think it's very much, if I can only manage twenty minutes, that's fine. I'm not going to beat myself up mentally that I haven't done enough. It's fine. I'll try and do more next time.'[13]

Kirk Erickson says that, for him, a lot of the battle is about simply remembering to move: 'I'm just like everyone else. I get engrossed, and piles of work get on my desk – I can't move for hours at a time. And so I have to remain very cognisant of my behaviours and make sure that I get up, take breaks, take lunch breaks where I take a good walk.' His leisure-based compensatory activity is to watch a Netflix series on an iPad while using a treadmill: 'We always need to find activities that we enjoy. Because if you start trying to do something because you know it's healthy, but you don't enjoy it, it's unlikely you're going to continue to adhere to it.'[14]

Jan Gehl says that even at the age of eighty-three he is nagged by his daughter, a doctor, to make sure he walks enough, even if he does not always manage the mandated 10,000 daily steps. 'No,' he admits. 'But I aim to be between 7,000 and 9,000. That's quite good. And it's easier when I travel. Heathrow airport will always give you 5,000 steps.'[15]

Steven Blair is marginally younger, at eighty, and says that his former activity as a keen if 'not very good' marathon runner has now turned into walking, as well as muscular resistance training. When he turned seventy, Blair set himself the ambitious target of walking 5 million steps a year, which averages out at just under 14,000 a day, which he has reached every year since. He sums up his approach like this: 'It's mainly doing something, and what will work for you. People ask, "What is the best activity to do?" And my simple-minded answer is, "The one you'll do and keep doing."[16]

Blair is, of course, being deliberately self-mocking. This is a man who has spent almost sixty years in academia, most of it at the vanguard of research into why people are inactive, how they can become more active, and what happens, on individual and population-wide levels, if they do not. He was the lead editor on the landmark 1996 US government report which effectively introduced inactivity to the global policy mainstream. And his words are very much at the heart of what, more than twenty-five years later, still needs to happen.

'Physical activity' is a technical term, and can feel slightly dry, almost joyless. This book is, I hope, instead more of a love letter to one of the most fundamental elements of what it means to be human – to be in motion, to exert yourself, to feel that natural yet almost inexpressible sensation as some of the 600-plus skeletal muscles in your body burn joyfully through their ever-replenishing stocks of adenosine triphosphate to do ... well, something. Anything.

It could be a walk around the block to a friend's house. It might be ascending a flight of stairs into work. Those fatigue-resistant leg muscles could be instead pedalling you across town to a meal with a loved one in a favourite restaurant. Your body might be engaged in a relatively sedate three METs of effort, or raising a brief sweat at ten or twelve, as you cycle up a hill. It matters not. We've already seen the endless benefits that come from using the human body, even occasionally, in the way it was intended through countless centuries of hunting, gathering, farming, strolling, leaping and playing. So how do you do more of it? For now, forget the gym, or the running shoes. Think instead about your day-to-day routine, and how movement fits into it, or how it perhaps could. This won't always be easy, and if so will most likely be caused by factors well beyond the control of you or any individual. But, somewhere, that physical routine, that daily exhilaration from being in motion, is there. So go out and find what it is. And then just keep doing it. It's really as simple as that.

ENDNOTES

Introduction

1 Inactivity statistics are collected separately by each UK nation, so the total figure is somewhat approximate.

  NHS Health Survey for England 2016: Physical Activity in Adults http://healthsurvey.hscic.gov.uk/media/63730/HSE16-Adult-phy-act.pdf

  Public Health Scotland: Physical Activity Overview http://www.healthscotland.scot/health-topics/physical-activity/physical-activity-overview#:~:text=Half%20of%20all%20adults%20aged,deaths%20in%20Scotland%20each%20year.

  Government of Wales: National Survey for Wales 2018–19, Adult Lifestyle https://gov.wales/sites/default/files/statistics-and-research/2019-06/national-survey-for-wales-april-2018-to-march-2019-adult-lifestyle-534.pdf

  Northern Ireland Health Survey: First Results (2016/17) https://www.health-ni.gov.uk/sites/default/files/publications/health/hsni-first-results-16-17.pdf

2 NHS Health Survey for England 2015: Physical Activity in Children http://healthsurvey.hscic.gov.uk/media/37752/hse2015-child-phy-act.pdf

3 Pedro C. Hallal et al., 'Global physical activity levels: surveillance progress, pitfalls, and prospects', *The Lancet*, Vol. 380, No. 9838 (2012): 247–57.

4 Sue Bowden, Avner Offer, 'Household appliances and the use of time: the United States and Britain since the 1920s', *Economic History Review*, Vol. 47, No. 4 (1994): 725–48.

5 David Kynaston, *Modernity Britain: Opening the Box 1957–59* (London: Bloomsbury, 2013), p. 61.

6 Office for National Statistics: Long-term trends in UK employment, 1861 to 2018. Chart using Bank of England historic data.

7 Figure provided by cycling author and historian Carlton Reid.
8 Department for Transport, National Travel Survey: England 2018. https://assets.publishing.service.gov.uk/government/uploads/system/uploads/attachment_data/file/823068/national-travel-survey-2018.pdf
9 Department for Transport, National Travel Survey: England 2018.
10 Public Health England: Research and analysis – Brisk walking and physical inactivity in 40- to 60-year-olds (June 2018).
11 National Travel Survey: England 2018.
12 Data from Active People Interactive research tool on Sport England website.
13 I-Min Lee et al., 'Effect of physical inactivity on major non-communicable diseases worldwide: an analysis of burden of disease and life expectancy', *The Lancet*, Vol. 380, No. 9838 (2012): 219–29.
14 Peace Research Institute Oslo: Trends in Armed Conflict, 1946–2018. It says about 53,000 died in war worldwide in 2018.
15 For example, NHS figures say about 78,000 people a year die in the UK because of tobacco, against an estimated 100,000 due to inactive living.
16 Public Health England, Physical activity: applying All Our Health (October 2019). This says inactivity is responsible for one in six UK deaths, and there are about 600,000 deaths per year across the UK.
17 Interview with the author.
18 Lars Bo Andersen et al., 'All-Cause Mortality Associated with Physical Activity During Leisure Time, Work, Sports, and Cycling to Work', *Archives of Internal Medicine*, Vol. 160, No. 11 (2000): 1621–8.
19 Statistic from Asthma UK.

Chapter 1

1 Timothy M. Ryan, Colin N. Shaw, 'Gracility of the modern *Homo sapiens* skeleton is the result of decreased biomechanical loading', *Proceedings of the National Academy of Sciences of the United States of America*, Vol. 112, No. 2 (2015): 372–7.
2 Jennifer M. Hootnam, 'Physical Activity, Fitness and Joint and Bone Health', in *Physical Activity and Health*, eds Claude Bouchard, Steven N. Blair, William L. Haskell (Champaign, Illinois: Human Kinetics, 2012), p. 247. Citing Arthritis Foundation research.
3 Alison A. Macintosh, Ron Pinhasi, Jay T. Stock, 'Prehistoric women's manual labor exceeded that of athletes through the first 5500 years of farming in Central Europe', *Science Advances*, Vol. 3, No. 11 (2017).
4 David R. Bassett Jr, Patrick L. Schneider, Gertrude E.

Endnotes

Huntingdon, 'Physical Activity in an Old Order Amish Community', *Medicine and Science in Sports and Exercise*, Vol. 36, No. 1 (2004): 79–85.

5 UK Data Service: Urban Population Database, 1801–1911 (Robert J. Bennett, University of Cambridge).

6 Lorraine Lanningham-Foster, Lana J. Nysse, James A. Levine, 'Labor Saved, Calories Lost: The Energetic Impact of Domestic Labor-saving Devices', *Obesity Research*, Vol. 11, No. 10 (2003): 1178–81.

7 NHS: What should my daily intake of calories be? https://www.nhs.uk/common-health-questions/food-and-diet/what-should-my-daily-intake-of-calories-be/

8 Physical Activity and Health – A Report of the Surgeon General (1996). https://www.cdc.gov/nccdphp/sgr/pdf/sgrfull.pdf

9 Interview with the author.

10 James S. Skinner, 'The Fitness Industry', in *The Academy Papers: Physical Activity in Early and Modern Populations*, eds Robert S. Malina, Helen M. Eckert (Champaign, Illinois: Human Kinetics Books, 1988).

11 NHS Health Survey for England 2016: Physical Activity in Adults

12 NHS Health Survey for England 2016: Physical Activity in Adults

13 Health Survey for England 2015: Physical Activity in Children http://healthsurvey.hscic.gov.uk/media/37752/hse2015-child-phy-act.pdf

14 Pamela Das, Richard Horton, 'Rethinking our approach to physical activity', *The Lancet*, Vol. 380, No. 9838 (2012): 189–90.

15 Pedro C. Hallal et al., 'Global physical activity levels: surveillance progress, pitfalls, and prospects', *The Lancet*, Vol. 380, No. 9838 (2012): 247–257.

16 Salomé Aubert et al., 'Global Matrix 3.0 Physical Activity Report Card Grades for Children and Youth: Results and Analysis From 49 Countries', *Journal of Physical Activity and Health*, Vol. 15, No. S2 (2018): S251–S273.

17 Shu Wen Ng, Barry Popkin, 'Time Use and Physical Activity: A Shift Away from Movement Across the Globe', *Obesity Reviews*, Vol. 13, No. 8 (2012): 659–80.

18 William L. Haskell, with Steven N. Blair and Claude Bouchard, 'An Integrated View of Physical Activity, Fitness and Health', in *Physical Activity and Health*, eds Claude Bouchard, Steven N. Blair, William L. Haskell (Champaign, Illinois: Human Kinetics, 2012), p. 415.

19 Carl J. Caspersen, Kenneth E. Powell, Gregory M. Christenson, 'Physical Activity, Exercise, and Physical Fitness: Definitions and Distinctions for Health-Related Research', *Public Health Reports*, Vol. 100, No. 2 (1985): 126–31.

20 Interview with the author.

21 Jennifer Smith Maguire, *Fit For Consumption: Sociology and the Business of Fitness* (Abingdon: Routledge, 2008).

22 Estimates for the size and revenues of the global fitness industry
    vary considerably: the figure of about £65 billion comes from the
    Health Club Management Handbook.
23 Olivia Zaleski, Kiel Porter, 'Peloton Picks Goldman Sachs,
    JPMorgan to Lead IPO', *Bloomberg News*, 25 February 2019.
24 Figures taken from the ultramarathon section of the Findarace
    .com website.
25 Statistics from 2019 State of the UK Fitness and Swimming
    Industry Report, by the Leisure Database Company.
26 Interview with the author.
27 Jo Ellison, 'The dumb-bell economy: inside the booming
    business of exercise', *Financial Times*, 9 February 2018.
28 UK Sport: Historical Funding Figures – Summer Olympics
    https://www.uksport.gov.uk/our-work/investing-in-sport/
    historical-funding-figures
29 Public Health England: Annual Report and Accounts 2018/19.
30 Active People Interactive research tool on Sport England website.
31 Department for Transport. National Travel Survey: England
    2018 (p. 2) https://assets.publishing.service.gov.uk/government/
    uploads/system/uploads/attachment_data/file/823068/national-
    travel-survey-2018.pdf
32 Active People Interactive research tool on Sport England website.
33 Stian Alexander, 'Brits wasting £558m on unused gym
    memberships – with 11% saying they haven't been in a year',
    Daily Mirror, 23 January 2017.
34 Interview with the author.

Chapter 2

1 Claude Bouchard, with Steven N. Blair and William L. Haskell,
   'Why Study Physical Activity, and Health?', in *Physical Activity
   and Health*, eds Claude Bouchard, Steven N. Blair, William L.
   Haskell (Champaign, Illinois: Human Kinetics, 2012), p. 4.
2 Matthew M. Robinson et al., 'Enhanced Protein Translation
   Underlies Improved Metabolic and Physical Adaptations to
   Different Exercise Training Modes in Young and Old Humans',
   Cell Metabolism, Vol. 25, No. 3 (2017): 581–92.
3 Zoë Corbyn, 'Elizabeth Blackburn on the telomere effect: "It's
   about keeping healthier for longer"', *The Observer*, 29 January
   2017.
4 Larry A. Tucker, 'Physical activity and telomere length in US men
   and women: An NHANES investigation', *Preventative Medicine*,
   Vol. 100 (2017): 145–51.
5 Natassa V. Tsetsonis, Adrienne E. Hardman, Sarabjit S. Mastana,
   'Acute effects of exercise on postprandial lipemia: a comparative
   study in trained and untrained middle-aged women', *American
   Journal of Clinical Nutrition*, Vol. 65, No. 2 (1997): 525–33.

6 Francine E. Garrett-Bakelman et al., 'The NASA Twins Study: A multidimensional analysis of a year-long human spaceflight', *Science*, Vol. 364, No. 6436 (2019): 127–8.

7 Interview with the author.

8 Updated edition: 2018 Physical Activity Guidelines Advisory Committee Scientific Report. Co-chairs of committee: Abby C. King and Kenneth E. Powell https://health.gov/sites/default/files/2019-09/PAG_Advisory_Committee_Report.pdf

9 Michael F. Leitzmann et al., 'Physical activity recommendations and decreased risk of mortality', *Archives of Internal Medicine*, Vol. 167, No. 22 (2007): 2453–60.

10 Steven N. Blair et al., 'Physical Fitness and All-Cause Mortality: A Prospective Study of Healthy Men and Women', *Journal of the American Medical Association*, Vol. 262, No. 17 (1989): 2395–401.

11 I. M. Lee et al., 'Effect of physical inactivity on major non-communicable diseases worldwide: an analysis of burden of disease and life expectancy,' *The Lancet*, Vol. 380, No. 9838 (2012): 219–29.

12 World Health Organization, Global Health Risks: Mortality and burden of disease attributable to selected major risks (2009). https://www.who.int/healthinfo/global_burden_disease/GlobalHealthRisks_report_full.pdf

13 I-Min Lee et al., 'Annual deaths attributable to physical inactivity: whither the missing 2 million?', Correspondence in *The Lancet*, Vol. 381, No. 9871 (2013): 992–3.

14 J. N. Morris, J. A. Heady, P. A. Raffle, C. G. Roberts, J. W. Parks, 'Coronary heart-disease and physical activity of work', *The Lancet*, Vol. 262, No. 6795 (1953): 1053–7.

15 Mihaela Tanasescu et al., 'Exercise Type and Intensity in Relation to Coronary Heart Disease in Men', *Journal of the American Medical Association*, Vol. 288, No. 16 (2002): 1994–2000.

16 2018 Physical Activity Guidelines Advisory Committee Scientific Report.

17 2018 Physical Activity Guidelines Advisory Committee Scientific Report.

18 Jaakko Tuomilehto et al., 'Prevention of Type 2 Diabetes Mellitus by Changes in Lifestyle among Subjects with Impaired Glucose Tolerance', *New England Journal of Medicine*, Vol. 344 (2001): 1343–50.

19 Statistics from the charity Age UK in 2013 https://www.ageuk.org.uk/latest-press/archive/250000-older-people-hospitalised-due-to-a-fall-every-year/

20 World Health Organization, Physical Activity and Adults https://www.who.int/dietphysicalactivity/factsheet_adults/en/

21 Interview with the author.

22 Interview with the author.

23 Catrine Tudor-Locke et al., 'How fast is fast enough? Walking cadence (steps/min) as a practical estimate of intensity in adults:

a narrative review', *British Journal of Sports Medicine*, Vol. 52, No. 12 (2018): 776–88.

24 Terence Dwyer et al., 'Objectively Measured Daily Steps and Subsequent Long Term All-Cause Mortality: The Tasped Prospective Cohort Study', *PLOS One*, Vol. 10, No. 11 (2015).

25 I-Min Lee et al., 'Association of Step Volume and Intensity with All-Cause Mortality in Older Women', *JAMA Internal Medicine*, Vol. 179, No. 8 (2019): 1105–12.

26 Interview with the author.

27 2018 Physical Activity Guidelines Advisory Committee Scientific Report.

28 Hmwe H. Kyu et al., 'Physical activity and risk of breast cancer, colon cancer, diabetes, ischemic heart disease, and ischemic stroke events: systematic review and dose-response meta-analysis for the Global Burden of Disease Study 2013', *British Medical Journal*, Vol. 354:i3857 (2016).

29 I-Min Lee, Howard D. Sesso, Yuko Oguma, Ralph S. Paffenbarger, Jr, 'The "Weekend Warrior" and Risk of Mortality', *American Journal of Epidemiology*, Vol. 160, No. 7 (2004): 636–41.

30 Gary O'Donovan, I-Min Lee et al., 'Association of "Weekend Warrior" and Other Leisure Time Physical Activity Patterns With Risks for All-Cause, Cardiovascular Disease, and Cancer Mortality', *JAMA Internal Medicine*, Vol. 177, No. 3 (2017): 335–42.

Chapter 3

1 William Buchan, *Domestic Medicine: or, a Treatise on the Prevention and Cure of Diseases by Regimen and Simple Medicines* (1769).

2 Carleton B. Chapman, 'Edward Smith (? 1818–1874) Physiologist, Human Ecologist, Reformer', *Journal of the History of Medicine and Allied Sciences*, Vol. 22, No. 1 (1967): 1–26.

3 Percival Horton-Smith Hartley, 'The Longevity of Oarsmen', *British Medical Journal*, 1:4082 (1939): 657–62.

4 Alan Rook, 'An Investigation into the Longevity of Cambridge Sportsmen', *British Medical Journal*, 1:4865 (1954): 773–7.

5 Family history by Joshua Plaut sent to the author.

6 Oxford Brookes University: Professor Jeremy Morris CBE FRCP in interview with Max Blythe (1986).
    Video: https://radar.brookes.ac.uk/radar/items/2d190b9a-e481-43e6-9956-5b39be502f63/1/
    Transcript: https://radar.brookes.ac.uk/radar/file/2d190b9a-e481-43e6-9956-5b39be502f63/1/Morris%2CJ.pdf

7 Simon Kuper, 'The man who invented exercise', *Financial Times*, 12 September 2009.

8 Interview with Max Blythe.

9 Interview with Max Blythe.

10 Interview with Max Blythe.

Endnotes

11 Geoff Watts, 'Exercising his passion – interview with Jerry Morris', *British Medical Journal*, Vol. 321, No. 7255 (2000): 198.

12 Kuper, 'The man who invented exercise'.

13 Jerry Morris, 'Physical activity versus heart attack: a modern epidemic – personal observations', in *Epidemiologic Methods in Physical Activity Studies*, ed. I-Min Lee (Oxford: Oxford University Press, 2008).

14 Interview with Max Blythe.

15 Kuper, 'The man who invented exercise'.

16 Morris, 'Physical activity versus heart attack: a modern epidemic – personal observations'.

17 Watts, 'Exercising his passion – interview with Jerry Morris'.

18 Kuper, 'The man who invented exercise'.

19 Kuper, 'The man who invented exercise'.

20 Interview with the author.

21 Hans Kraus, Wilhelm Raab, *Hypokinetic Disease: Diseases Caused by Lack of Exercise* (Springfield, Illinois: Thomas, 1961).

22 Ralph S. Paffenbarger Jr et al., 'Work activity of longshoremen as related to death from coronary heart disease and stroke', *New England Journal of Medicine*, Vol. 282, No. 20 (1970): 1109–14.

23 Ralph S. Paffenbarger Jr, Alvin L. Wing, Robert T. Hyde, 'Physical activity as an index of heart attack risk in college alumni', *American Journal of Epidemiology*, Vol. 108, No. 3 (1978): 161–75.

24 Ralph S. Paffenbarger Jr, Robert T. Hyde, Chung-Cheng Hsieh, Alvin L. Wing, 'Physical Activity, Other Life-style Patterns, Cardiovascular Disease and Longevity', *Acta Medica Scandinavica*, Vol. 220, No. S711 (1986): 85–91.

25 The *Women's Health Study*, a long-term study of nurses and other health professionals in the US and Puerto Rico.

26 Interview with the author.

27 Interview from 1996 by Associated Press, quoted in Valerie J. Nelson, 'Dr. Ralph Paffenbarger, 84; linked exercise, longevity in influential study', *Los Angeles Times*, 16 July 2007.

28 Jeremy Pearce, 'R. S. Paffenbarger Jr., 84, Epidemiologist, Dies', *New York Times*, 14 July 2007.

29 Kenneth H. Cooper, *Aerobics* (New York: M. Evans & Company, 1968).

30 Amby Burfoot, 'RIP – Dr. Ralph Paffenbarger (1922–2007), Friend, Ultramarathoner, Fitness Pioneer', *Runner's World*, 12 July 2007.

31 V. Berridge, A. Mold, 'Jerry Morris memorial conference', *Public Health*, Vol. 125, No. 3 (2011): 172–3.

32 Kuper, 'The man who invented exercise'.

33 Interview with the author.

34 Interview with the author.

35 Watts, 'Exercising his passion – interview with Jerry Morris'.

36 Kuper, 'The man who invented exercise'.

37 I-Min Lee, Charles E. Matthews, Steven N. Blair, 'The Legacy of Dr. Ralph Seal Paffenbarger, Jr. – Past, Present, and Future

Contributions to Physical Activity Research', *President's Council on Physical Fitness and Sports Research Digest*, Vol. 10, No. 1 (2009): 1–8.

38 Author's interview with I-Min Lee.

39 Kuper, 'The man who invented exercise'.

40 Virginia Berridge, 'Celebration: Jerry Morris', *International Journal of Epidemiology*, Vol. 30, No. 5 (2001): 1141–5.

41 Interview with the author.

42 Interview with the author.

43 Jerry Morris (chair of investigator), *Allied Dunbar National Fitness Survey* (Health Education Authority/Sports Council, 1990).

44 Kuper, 'The man who invented exercise'.

45 Dennis Hevesi, 'Jeremy Morris, Who Proved Exercise Is Heart-Healthy, Dies at 99½', *New York Times*, 7 November 2009.

46 Ann Oakley, 'Appreciation: Jerry [Jeremiah Noah] Morris, 1910–2009', *International Journal of Epidemiology*, Vol. 39, No. 1 (2010): 274–6.

Chapter 4

1 Interview with the author.

2 The King's Fund, 'Data briefing: why NHS budgets have always been a bugbear', February 2008 https://www.kingsfund.org.uk/publications/articles/data-briefing-why-nhs-budgets-have-always-been-bugbear

3 NHS England, 2018/19 Annual report, p9 https://www.england.nhs.uk/wp-content/uploads/2019/07/Annual-Report-Full-201819.pdf

4 Office for National Statistics, 'How has life expectancy changed over time?', 9 September 2015 https://www.ons.gov.uk/peoplepopulationandcommunity/birthsdeathsandmarriages/lifeexpectancies/articles/howhaslifeexpectancychangedovertime/2015-09-09

5 Royal College of Physicians, 'Fifty years since *Smoking and Health*: Progress, lessons and priorities for a smoke-free UK', March 2012: p vii https://www.rcplondon.ac.uk/file/2547/download

6 British Heart Foundation, 'UK Factsheet: July 2020' https://www.bhf.org.uk/-/media/files/research/heart-statistics/bhf-cvd-statistics-uk-factsheet.pdf?la=en

7 Office for National Statistics, 'National life tables, UK: 2016 to 2018' https://www.ons.gov.uk/peoplepopulationandcommunity/birthsdeathsandmarriages/lifeexpectancies/bulletins/nationallifetablesunitedkingdom/2016to2018

8 Office for National Statistics, 'Health state life expectancies, UK: 2015 to 2017' https://www.ons.gov.uk/peoplepopulationandcommunity/

healthandsocialcare/healthandlifeexpectancies/bulletins/
healthstatelifeexpectanciesuk/2015to2017

9   Office for National Statistics, 'General Lifestyle Survey Overview –
    a report on the 2011 General Lifestyle Survey – Chapter 7', March
    2013 https://www.ons.gov.uk/peoplepopulationandcommunity/
    personalandhouseholdfinances/incomeandwealth/compendium/
    generallifestylesurvey/2013-03-07

10 Age UK, 'Later Life in the United Kingdom 2019' https://www
    .ageuk.org.uk/globalassets/age-uk/documents/reports-and-
    publications/later_life_uk_factsheet.pdf

11 Interview with the author.

12 Diabetes UK, 'Tackling the crisis: Transforming diabetes care
    for a better future – England' https://www.diabetes.org.uk/
    resources-s3/2019-04/Diabetes%20UK%20Tackling%20the%20
    Crisis.pdf

13 Diabetes UK estimates 4.7 million people in the UK have
    diabetes, with 90% of these having diabetes type 2. Diabetes
    UK fact sheet https://www.diabetes.org.uk/resources-s3/2019-
    02/1362B_Facts%20and%20stats%20Update%20Jan%20
    2019_LOW%20RES_EXTERNAL.pdf

14 Diabetes UK, 'The cost of diabetes', 2017 https://www.diabetes
    .org.uk/resources-s3/2017-11/diabetes%20uk%20cost%20of%20
    diabetes%20report.pdf

15 Diabetes UK, 'Nearly 7,000 children and young adults with
    Type 2 diabetes', November 2018 https://www.diabetes.org.uk/
    about-us/news/children-young-adults-type-2-rise

16 Public Health England, 'Physical inactivity: economic costs to
    NHS clinical commissioning groups', April 2016 https://assets
    .publishing.service.gov.uk/government/uploads/system/uploads/
    attachment_data/file/524234/Physical_inactivity_costs_to_CCGs
    .pdf

17 Estimated cost is $131 billion, before adjusting for BMI, and $117
    billion after; Susan A. Carlson, Janet E. Fulton, Michael Pratt,
    Zhou Yang, E. Kathleen Adams, 'Inadequate Physical Activity
    and Health Care Expenditures in the United States', *Progress in
    Cardiovascular Diseases*, Vol. 57, No. 4 (2015): 315–23.

18 Ding Ding et al., 'The economic burden of physical inactivity: a
    global analysis of major non-communicable diseases', *The Lancet*,
    Vol. 388, No. 10051 (2016): 1311–24.

19 Interview with the author.

20 Interview with the author.

21 Patrick Butler, 'Tory county council runs out of cash to meet
    obligations', *The Guardian*, 3 February 2018.

22 Interview with the author.

23 Marco Pahor et al., 'Effect of structured physical activity on
    prevention of major mobility disability in older adults: the LIFE
    Study randomized clinical trial', *Journal of the American Medical
    Association*, Vol. 311, No. 23 (2014): 2387–96.

24 NHS Long Term Plan https://www.longtermplan.nhs.uk/
25 Interview with the author.

Chapter 5

1 Jan Gehl, translated from the Danish by Jo Koch, *Life Between Buildings* (Washington DC: Island Press, originally published 1971, this edition 2006).
2 Interview with the author.
3 United Nations Department of Economic and Social Affairs, 'World Urbanization Prospects 2018' https://population.un.org/wup/Publications/Files/WUP2018-Highlights.pdf
4 Mark Easton, 'Five mind-blowing facts about what the UK looks like', *BBC News*, 9 November 2017.
5 Department for Environment and Rural Affairs, 'Official Statistics: Rural population 2014/15, Updated 27 August 2020' https://www.gov.uk/government/publications/rural-population-and-migration/rural-population-201415
6 Carlos A Celis-Morales et al., 'Association between active commuting and incident cardiovascular disease, cancer, and mortality: prospective cohort study', *British Medical Journal*, Vol. 357, No. 1456 (2017).
7 Andersen et al., 'All-Cause Mortality Associated with Physical Activity During Leisure Time, Work, Sports, and Cycling to Work'.
8 Public Health England. Physical activity: applying All Our Health (October 2019).
9 In 2018 there were ninety-nine cyclist fatalities; Department for Transport, 'Reported road casualties in Great Britain: 2018 annual report' https://assets.publishing.service.gov.uk/government/uploads/system/uploads/attachment_data/file/834585/reported-road-casualties-annual-report-2018.pdf
10 The calculation is approximate, as it depends how you measure it. One 2012 study (see reference below) calculated that cycling in the UK was 3.4 times more dangerous than in the Netherlands, based on deaths per million hours ridden. But Professor Rachel Aldred, an expert on cycling from Westminster University, has taken these figures and factored in the higher numbers of older people who cycle in the Netherlands, and the greater chance of death they face due to complications from injuries like broken bones (in the Netherlands if someone dies within thirty days of a traffic incident, it is marked down as a road death). On this basis, she estimated cycling in the UK is just over four times as dangerous; Jennifer Mindell, Deborah Leslie, Malcolm Wardlaw, 'Exposure-Based, "Like-for-Like" Assessment of Road Safety by Travel Mode Using Routine Health Data,' PLOS One, Vol. 7, No. 12 (2012).

Endnotes

11 Jeroen Johan De Hartog, Hanna Boogaard, Hans Nijland, Gerard Hoek, 'Do the Health Benefits of Cycling Outweigh the Risks?' *Environmental Health Perspectives*, Vol. 118, No. 8 (2010): 1109–16.

12 Rachel Aldred et al., 'Cycling Near Misses: Findings from Year One of the Near Miss Project,' 2015 http://rachelaldred.org/wp-content/uploads/2019/03/Nearmissreport-final-web.pdf

13 Analysis by Professor Rachel Aldred of Westminster University for her 'Project Pedestrian' study. It found that 548 pedestrians were killed in the UK on pavements or verges between 2005 and 2018.

14 Peter Walker, 'Reduction in passenger road deaths "not matched by cyclists and pedestrians"', *The Guardian*, 30 January 2020.

15 Colin Buchanan, *Traffic in Towns* (London: Penguin, 1964).

16 Vic Langenhoff, Stop de Kindermoord, *De Tijd*, 20 September 1972. Langenhoff wrote the article after his daughter Simone had been killed by a speeding car. The driver was fined the equivalent of £20. Then one of his older daughters was injured after being forced off her bike by a driver. Langenhoff said his new pressure group would try and 'break through the apathy with which the Dutch people accept the daily carnage of children in traffic', writing: 'This country chooses one kilometre of motorway over 100 kilometres of safe cycle paths. There's no pressure group? Let's start one. Parents of little victims, worried parents of potential little victims: unite.'

17 Takemi Sugiyama et al., 'Neighborhood Walkability and TV Viewing Time Among Australian Adults', *American Journal of Preventive Medicine*, Vol. 33, No. 6 (2007): 444–9.

18 Alison Carver et al., 'How are the built environment and household travel characteristics associated with children's active transport in Melbourne, Australia?', *Journal of Transport and Health*, Vol. 12 (2019): 115–29.

19 Gehl, *Life Between Buildings*.

20 David Sim, *Soft City: Building Density for Everyday Life* (Washington DC: Island Press, 2019).

21 Interview with the author.

22 Peter Walker, 'Utrecht's Cycling Lessons for Migrants: "Riding a Bike Makes Me Feel More Dutch"', *The Guardian*, 28 April 2016.

23 CROW, 'Design manual for bicycle traffic', 2007 https://www.crow.nl/publicaties/design-manual-for-bicycle-traffic

24 Mark Wagenbuur, 'Dutch cycling figures', *Bicycle Dutch*, January 2018 https://bicycledutch.wordpress.com/2018/01/02/dutch-cycling-figures/

25 Department for Transport, National Travel Survey 2018.

26 2011 Census: distance travelled to work.

27 Pedro C. Hallal et al., 'Global physical activity levels: surveillance progress, pitfalls, and prospects', *The Lancet*, Vol. 380, No. 9838 (2012): 247–57.

28 Bike Europe, 'E-Bike Now Biggest Category in the Netherlands', 5

March 2019 https://www.bike-eu.com/market/nieuws/2019/03/e-bike-now-biggest-category-in-the-netherlands-10135442

29 Alberto Castro et al., 'Physical activity of electric bicycle users compared to conventional bicycle users and non-cyclists: Insights based on health and transport data from an online survey in seven European cities', *Transportation Research Interdisciplinary Perspectives*, Vol. 1 (2019).

30 Interview with the author.

31 All statistics from Odense municipality.

32 Interview with the author.

33 Avril Blamey, Nanette Mutrie, Tom Aitchison, 'Health promotion by encouraged use of stairs', *British Medical Journal*, Vol. 311, No. 7000 (1995): 289–90.

34 Juan Pablo Rey-Lopez, Emmanuel Stamatakisa, Martin Mackey, Howard D. Sessode, I-Min Lee, 'Associations of self-reported stair climbing with all-cause and cardiovascular mortality: The Harvard Alumni Health Study', *Preventative Medicine Reports*, Vol. 15 (2019).

35 Interview with the author.

36 Interview with the author.

37 Naoko Muramatsu, Hiroko Akiyama, 'Japan: Super-Aging Society Preparing for the Future', *The Gerontologist*, Vol. 51, No. 4 (2011): 425–32.

38 Bjarke Ingels Group, BIG leadership https://big.dk/#about

39 Interview with the author.

40 Caroline Criado-Perez, *Invisible Women: Exposing Data Bias in a World Designed for Men* (London: Vintage, 2020).

41 Data from Active People Interactive research tool on Sport England website.

Chapter 6

1 Interview with the author.

2 Tom Watson, *Downsizing: How I lost 8 stone, reversed my diabetes and regained my health* (London: Octopus, 2020).

3 Thomas Burgoine, Nita G, Forouhi, Simon J. Griffin, Nicholas J, Wareham, Pablo Monsivais, 'Associations between exposure to takeaway food outlets, takeaway food consumption, and body weight in Cambridgeshire, UK: population based, cross sectional study', *British Medical Journal*, Vol. 348 (2014): g1464.

4 Natasha A. Schvey et al., 'The Experience of Weight Stigma Among Gym Members with Overweight and Obesity', *Stigma and Health*, Vol. 2, No. 4 (2017): 292–306.

5 Interview with the author.

6 Iris Shai et al., 'Ethnicity, obesity, and risk of type 2 diabetes in women: a 20-year follow-up study', *Diabetes Care*, Vol. 29, No. 7 (2006): 1585–90.

Endnotes

7 Paul Deurenberg, Mabel Deurenberg-Yap, Syafri Guricci, 'Asians are different from Caucasians and from each other in their body mass index/body fat per cent relationship', *Obesity Reviews*, Vol. 3 (2002): 141-6.

8 World Health Organization expert consultation, 'Appropriate body-mass index for Asian populations and its implications for policy and intervention strategies', *The Lancet*, Vol. 363 (2004) https://www.who.int/nutrition/publications/bmi_asia_strategies.pdf?ua=1; https://www.gov.scot/publications/obesity-indicators/pages/4/

9 NHS: Health Survey for England 2018. Overweight and obesity in adults and children, December 2019 https://files.digital.nhs.uk/52/FD7E18/HSE18-Adult-Child-Obesity-rep.pdf

10 Scottish government: Obesity Indicators 2018.

11 Health Survey for England 2018.

12 Health Survey for England 2018.

13 Health Survey for England 2018.

14 World Health Organization, 'Factsheets: Obesity and overweight', April 2020 https://www.who.int/news-room/fact-sheets/detail/obesity-and-overweight

15 Dr Margaret Chan, 'Obesity and diabetes: the slow-motion disaster – Keynote address at the 47th meeting of the National Academy of Medicine', Washington DC, 17 October 2016 https://www.who.int/dg/speeches/2016/obesity-diabetes-disaster/en/

16 Marie Ng et al., 'Global, regional, and national prevalence of overweight and obesity in children and adults during 1980–2013: a systematic analysis for the Global Burden of Disease Study 2013', *The Lancet*, Vol. 384, No. 9945 (2014): 766–81.

17 Youfa Wang et al., 'Prevention and control of obesity in China', *The Lancet Global Health*, Vol. 7, No. 9 (2019): E1166–E1167.

18 Rajeev Ahirwar, Prakash Ranjan Mondal, 'Prevalence of obesity in India: A systematic review', *Diabetes and Metabolic Syndrome: Clinical Research and Reviews*, Vol. 13, No. 1 (2019): 318–32.

19 NHS: Statistics on Obesity, Physical Activity and Diet, England, 2019 (May 2019) https://digital.nhs.uk/data-and-information/publications/statistical/statistics-on-obesity-physical-activity-and-diet/statistics-on-obesity-physical-activity-and-diet-england-2019/part-1-obesity-related-hospital-admissions

20 Sarah Boseley, 'Global cost of obesity-related illness to hit $1.2tn a year from 2025', *The Guardian*, 10 October 2017.

21 Stanley N. Gershoff, 'Jean Mayer: 1920–1993', *Journal of Nutrition*, Vol. 131, No. 6 (2001): 1651–4.

22 Jean Mayer, 'The physiological basis of obesity and leanness I', *Nutrition Abstracts and Reviews*, Vol. 25, No. 3 (1955): 597–611.

23 Drew Desilver, 'What's on your table? How America's diet has changed over the decades', *Pew Research Center*, 13 December 2016.

24 Rachel Griffith, Rodrigo Lluberas, Melanie Lührmann, 'Gluttony

and Sloth? Calories, Labor Market Activity and the Rise of Obesity', *Journal of the European Economic Association*, Vol. 14, No. 6 (2016): 1253–86.

25 Katy Askew, 'Britons underestimate calorie intake by one third', *Food Navigator*, 18 February 2018.

26 Robert Ross, Ian Janssen, 'Physical Activity, Fitness and Obesity', in *Physical Activity and Health*, eds Claude Bouchard, Steven N. Blair, William L. Haskell (Champaign, Illinois; Human Kinetics, 2012), p. 205.

27 R. James Stubbs et al., 'A decrease in physical activity affects appetite, energy, and nutrient balance in lean men feeding ad libitum', *American Journal of Clinical Nutrition*, Vol. 79, No. 1 (2004): 62–9.

28 Stephen Whybrow et al., 'The effect of an incremental increase in exercise on appetite, eating behaviour and energy balance in lean men and women feeding *ad libitum*', *British Journal of Nutrition*, Vol. 100, No. 5 (2008): 1109–15.

29 Robert Ross, 'Physical Activity, Fitness and Obesity', in *Physical Activity and Health*, eds Claude Bouchard, Steven N. Blair, William L. Haskell (Champaign, Illinois: Human Kinetics, 2012), p. 200.

30 Dawn E. Alley, Virginia W. Chang, 'The Changing Relationship of Obesity and Disability, 1988–2004', *Journal of the American Medical Association*, Vol. 298, No. 17 (2007): 2020–7.

31 Flurin Item, Daniel Konrad, 'Visceral fat and metabolic inflammation: the portal theory revisited', *Obesity Review*, Vol. 13, No. S2 (2012): 30–9.

32 Robert Ross et al., 'Waist circumference as a vital sign in clinical practice: a Consensus Statement from the IAS and ICCR Working Group on Visceral Obesity', *Nature Reviews Endocrinology*, Vol. 16, No. 3 (2020): 177–89.

33 Interview with the author.

34 Diabetes UK: Diabetes Prevalence, January 2019 https://www.diabetes.co.uk/diabetes-prevalence.html

35 Silke Feller, Heiner Boeing, Tobias Pischon, 'Body Mass Index, Waist Circumference, and the Risk of Type 2 Diabetes Mellitus: Implications for Routine Clinical Practice', *Deutsches Ärzteblatt International*, Vol. 107, No. 26 (2010).

36 James R. Cerhan et al., 'A pooled analysis of waist circumference and mortality in 650,000 adults', *Mayo Clinic Proceedings*, Vol. 89, No. 3 (2014): 335–45.

37 Michael Lean et al., 'Waist circumference as a measure for indicating need for weight management', *British Medical Journal*, Vol. 311, No. 6998 (1995): 158–61.

38 NHS: Why is my waist size important? https://www.nhs.uk/common-health-questions/lifestyle/why-is-my-waist-size-important/

39 Win Saris et al., 'How much physical activity is enough to

prevent unhealthy weight gain? Outcome of the IASO 1st Stock Conference and consensus statement', *Obesity Reviews*, Vol. 4, No. 2 (2003): 101–14.

40 I Hadjiolova et al., 'Physical working capacity in obese women after an exercise programme for body weight reduction', *International Journal of Obesity*, Vol. 6 (1982): 405–10.

41 Naomi Y. J. Brinkmans et al., 'Energy expenditure and dietary intake in professional football players in the Dutch Premier League: Implications for nutritional counselling', *Journal of Sports Science*, Vol. 37, No. 24 (2019): 2759–67.

42 Interview with the author.

43 Chong Do Lee, Steven N. Blair, Andrew S. Jackson, 'Cardiorespiratory fitness, body composition, and all-cause and cardiovascular disease mortality in men', *American Journal of Clinical Nutrition*, Vol. 69, No. 3 (1999): 373–80.

44 Xuemei Sui, Steven N. Blair et al., 'Cardiorespiratory Fitness and Adiposity as Mortality Predictors in Older Adults', *Journal of the American Medical Association*, Vol. 298, No. 1 (2007): 2507–16.

45 Interview with the author.

46 Frank B. Hu et al., 'Adiposity as compared with physical activity in predicting mortality among women', *New England Journal of Medicine*, Vol. 351, No. 26 (2004): 2694–703.

47 ZiMian Wang et al., 'Systematic organization of body-composition methodology: an overview with emphasis on component-based methods', *American Journal of Clinical Nutrition*, Vol. 61, No. 3 (1995): 457–65.

Chapter 7

1 Calculation based on England, where there are about 7 million smokers (15% of an adult population of just over 47 million) and about 70,000 tobacco-related deaths per year. Smoking rates and deaths from NHS: Statistics on Smoking – England, 2018 https://digital.nhs.uk/data-and-information/publications/statistical/statistics-on-smoking/statistics-on-smoking-england-2018/

2 Neville Owen et al., 'Sedentary Behavior and Public Health: Integrating the Evidence and Identifying Potential Solutions', *Annual Review of Public Health*, Vol. 41 (2020): 265–87.

3 Maedeh Mansoubi et al., 'Energy expenditure during common sitting and standing tasks: examining the 1.5 MET definition of sedentary behaviour', *BMC Public Health*, Vol. 15, No. 1 (2015): 516.

4 Vybarr Cregan-Reid, *Primate Change* (London: Cassell, 2018), p. 12.

5 Cregan-Reid, *Primate Change*, p. 192–3.

6 Census figures compiled by Marjie Bloy, University of Singapore https://sites.google.com/site/motman/Home/information/occupations

7 NHS England: Why we should sit less https://www.nhs.uk/ live-well/exercise/why-sitting-too-much-is-bad-for-us/

8 Baker Heart and Diabetes Institute, What is sedentary behaviour? https://baker.edu.au/health-hub/rise-recharge

9 Adrian Bauman et al., 'The Descriptive Epidemiology of Sitting: A 20-Country Comparison Using the International Physical Activity Questionnaire (IPAQ)', *American Journal of Preventive Medicine*, Vol. 41, No. 2 (2011): 228–35.

10 Keith M. Diaz et al., 'Patterns of Sedentary Behavior in US Middle-Age and Older Adults: The REGARDS Study', *Medicine and Science in Sports and Exercise*, Vol. 48, No. 3 (2017): 430–8.

11 Officially known as the Sens Motion https://sens.dk/

12 Lionel Bey and Marc T. Hamilton, 'Suppression of skeletal muscle lipoprotein lipase activity during physical inactivity: a molecular reason to maintain daily low-intensity activity', *The Journal of Physiology*, Vol. 551, No. 2 (2003): 673–82.

13 B. Saltin, G. Blomqvist, J. H. Mitchell, R. L. Johnson Jr, K. Wildenthal, C. B. Chapman, 'Response to exercise after bed rest and after training', *Circulation*, Vol. 38, No. 5s7 (1968).

14 Alpa V. Patel et al., 'Prolonged Leisure Time Spent Sitting in Relation to Cause-Specific Mortality in a Large US Cohort', *American Journal of Epidemiology*, Vol. 187, No. 10 (2018): 2151–8.

15 Katrien Wijndaele et al., 'Television viewing time independently predicts all-cause and cardiovascular mortality: the EPIC Norfolk Study', *International Journal of Epidemiology*, Vol. 40, No. 1 (2011): 150–9.

16 Sarah K. Keadle et al., 'Causes of Death Associated with Prolonged TV Viewing', *American Journal of Preventive Medicine*, Vol. 49, No. 6 (2015): 811–21.

17 Interview with the author.

18 Cregan-Reid, *Primate Change*, p. 115.

19 Madina Saidj et al., 'Work and leisure time sitting and inactivity: Effects on cardiorespiratory and metabolic health', *European Journal of Preventive Cardiology*, Vol. 23, No. 12 (2015): 1321–9.

20 Mats Hallgren et al., 'Cross-sectional and prospective relationships of passive and mentally active sedentary behaviours and physical activity with depression', *British Journal of Psychiatry*, Vol. 217, No. 2 (2020): 413–19.

21 James Levine, *Get Up! Why Your Chair is Killing You and What You Can Do About it* (New York: St Martin's Griffin, 2014).

22 Levine, *Get Up!*, p. 39.

23 James A. Levine, Norman L. Eberhardt, Michael D. Jensen, 'Role of nonexercise activity thermogenesis in resistance to fat gain in humans', *Science*, Vol. 283, No. 5399 (1999): 212–14.

24 James A. Levine, Sara J. Schleusner, Michael D. Jensen, 'Energy expenditure of nonexercise activity', *American Journal of Clinical Nutrition*, Vol. 72, No. 6 (2000): 1451–4.

25 Ying Zhang et al., 'Basal metabolic rate of overweight and obese

adults in Beijing', *Wei Sheng Yan Jiu (Journal of Hygiene Research)*, Vol. 45, No. 5 (2016): 739–48.

26 Interview with the author.

27 Snehal M. Pinto Pereira, Myung Ki, Chris Power, 'Sedentary Behaviour and Biomarkers for Cardiovascular Disease and Diabetes in Mid-Life: The Role of Television-Viewing and Sitting at Work', *PLOS One*, Vol. 7, No. 2 (2012): Article e31132.

28 Patrik Wennberg, Per E. Gustafsson, David W. Dunstan, Maria Wennberg, Anne Hammarström, 'Television Viewing and Low Leisure-Time Physical Activity in Adolescence Independently Predict the Metabolic Syndrome in Mid-Adulthood', *Diabetes Care*, Vol. 36, No. 7 (2013): 2090–7.

29 Interview with the author.

30 Genevieve N. Healy et al., 'Breaks in Sedentary Time: Beneficial associations with metabolic risk', *Diabetes Care*, Vol. 31, No. 4 (2008): 661–6.

31 Keith M. Diaz et al., 'Patterns of Sedentary Behavior and Mortality in U.S. Middle-Aged and Older Adults: A National Cohort Study', *Annals of Internal Medicine*, Vol. 167, No. 7 (2017): 465–75.

32 Joseph Henson et al., 'Predictors of the acute postprandial response to breaking up prolonged sitting', *Medicine and Science in Sports and Exercise*, Vol. 52, No. 6 (2020): 1385–93.

33 Interview with the author.

34 Genevieve N. Healy et al., 'A Cluster Randomized Controlled Trial to Reduce Office Workers' Sitting Time: Effect on Activity Outcomes', *Medicine and Science in Sports and Exercise*, Vol. 48, No. 9 (2016): 1787–97.

35 Interview with the author.

36 Interview with the author.

37 Ulf Ekelund et al., 'Does physical activity attenuate, or even eliminate, the detrimental association of sitting time with mortality? A harmonised meta-analysis of data from more than 1 million men and women', *The Lancet*, Vol. 388, No. 10051 (2016): 1302–10.

38 Email correspondence with the author.

Chapter 8

1 Interview with the author.

2 Statistics supplied by Daily Mile.

3 NHS Health Survey for England 2016: Physical Activity in Adults.

4 NHS Health Survey for England 2015: Physical Activity in Children.

5 Hallal et al., 'Global physical activity levels: surveillance progress, pitfalls, and prospects'.

6 Gavin R. H. Sandercock, Ayodele Ogunleye, Christine Voss, 'Six

year changes in body mass index and cardiorespiratory fitness of English schoolchildren from an affluent area', *International Journal of Obesity*, Vol. 39, No. 10 (2015): 1504–7.

7 Gavin R. H. Sandercock, Daniel D. Cohen, 'Temporal trends in muscular fitness of English 10-year-olds 1998–2014: An allometric approach', *Journal of Science and Medicine in Sport*, Vol. 22, No. 2 (2019): 201–5.

8 Mark S, Tremblay, Joel D. Barnes, Jennifer L. Copeland, Dale W. Esliger, 'Conquering Childhood Inactivity: Is the Answer in the Past?', *Medicine and Science in Sports and Exercise*, Vol. 37, No. 7 (2005): 1187–94.

9 Finn Vejlø Rasmussen, Jess Lambrechtsen, Hans Christian Siersted, Henrik Steen Hansen, Neil C. Hansen, 'Low physical fitness in childhood is associated with the development of asthma in young adulthood: the Odense schoolchild study', *European Respiratory Journal*, Vol. 16, No. 5 (2000): 866–70.

10 John R. Mosley, 'Osteoporosis and bone functional adaptation: mechanobiological regulation of bone architecture in growing and adult bone, a review', *Journal of Rehabilitation Research and Development*, Vol. 37, No. 2 (2000): 189–99.

11 Regina Guthold, Gretchen A. Stevens, Leanne M. Riley, Fiona C. Bull, 'Global trends in insufficient physical activity among adolescents: a pooled analysis of 298 population-based surveys with 1.6 million participants', *The Lancet Child and Adolescent Health*, Vol. 4, No. 1 (2020): 23–35.

12 Health Education Authority, *Physical Activity at Our Time* (London: Health Education Authority, 2000).

13 Jay Coakley, Anita White, 'Making decisions: gender and sport participation among British adolescents', *Sociology of Sport Journal*, Vol. 9, No. 1 (1992): 20–35.

14 Guthold et al., 'Global trends in insufficient physical activity among adolescents'.

15 Department for Education national curriculums for primary and secondary schools.

16 Ofsted, 'Obesity, healthy eating and physical activity in primary schools', July 2018 https://assets.publishing.service.gov.uk/government/uploads/system/uploads/attachment_data/file/726114/Obesity__healthy_eating_and_physical_activity_in_primary_schools_170718.pdf

17 Scottish government, 'Health and wellbeing in schools' https://www.gov.scot/policies/schools/wellbeing-in-schools/

18 Neville Owen et al., 'Sedentary Behavior and Public Health: Integrating the Evidence and Identifying Potential Solutions', *Annual Review of Public Health*, Vol. 41 (2020): 265–87.

19 Diabetes UK, 'Nearly 7,000 children and young adults with Type 2 diabetes'.

20 Department for Transport, 'National Travel Survey 2014: Travel to School' https://assets.publishing.service.gov.uk/government/

uploads/system/uploads/attachment_data/file/476635/travel-to-school.pdf

21 Hidde P. van der Ploeg, Dafna Merom, Grace Corpuz, Adrian E. Bauman, 'Trends in Australian children traveling to school 1971–2003: Burning petrol or carbohydrates?', *Preventive Medicine*, Vol. 46, No. 1 (2008): 60–2.

22 Unicef, 'Child and adolescent injuries' https://www.unicef.org/health/injuries

23 Department for Transport, 'National Travel Survey 2014: Travel to School'.

24 Mathew Thomson, *Lost Freedom: The Landscape of the Child and the British Post-War Settlement* (Oxford: OUP, 2013), p. 141.

25 Department for Transport, 'Facts on child casualties: June 2015' https://assets.publishing.service.gov.uk/government/uploads/system/uploads/attachment_data/file/442236/child-casualties-2013-data.pdf

26 Department for Transport, 'Reported road casualties in Great Britain: 2018'.

27 Mayer Hillman, John Adams, John Whitelegg, *One False Move: A Study of Children's Independent Mobility* (London: Policy Studies Institute, 1990).

28 Leslie M. Alexander et al., 'The broader impact of walking to school among adolescents: seven day accelerometry based study', *British Medical Journal*, Vol. 331, No. 7524 (2005): 1061–2.

29 Interview with the author.

30 Tim Gill, *No Fear: Growing Up In A Risk-Averse Society* (London: Calouste Gulbenkian Foundation, 2007).

31 NHS Health Survey for England 2016: Physical Activity in Adults.

32 NHS: Exercise as you get older https://www.nhs.uk/live-well/exercise/exercise-as-you-get-older/

33 Office for National Statistics, Life Expectancies https://www.ons.gov.uk/peoplepopulationandcommunity/birthsdeathsandmarriages/lifeexpectancies

34 Office for National Statistics, Estimates of the very old, including centenarians, UK: 2002 to 2018 https://www.ons.gov.uk/peoplepopulationandcommunity/birthsdeathsandmarriages/ageing/bulletins/estimatesoftheveryoldincludingcentenarians/2002to2018#population-growth-of-those-aged-90-years-and-over-continues-to-decrease

35 Office for National Statistics, Health state life expectancies, UK: 2015 to 2017.

36 Neil McCartney, Stuart M. Phillips, 'Physical Activity, Muscular Fitness and Health', in *Physical Activity and Health*, eds Claude Bouchard, Steven N. Blair, William L. Haskell (Champaign, Illinois: Human Kinetics, 2012), p. 264.

37 This is the same for Public Health England, World Health Organization etc.

38 Patrick N. Siparsky, Donald T. Kirkendall, William E. Garrett Jr,

'Muscle Changes in Aging: Understanding Sarcopenia', *Sports Health*, Vol. 6, No. 1 (2014): 36–40.

39 NHS: Arthritis https://www.nhs.uk/conditions/arthritis/
40 US Department of Health and Human Services, 'Physical Activity Guidelines for Americans, Second Edition', 2018 https://health.gov/sites/default/files/2019-09/Physical_Activity_Guidelines_2nd_edition.pdf
41 NHS: Exercise https://www.nhs.uk/live-well/exercise/
42 Mie Tymn, 'John Keston: Age Group Ace', *Runner's World*, 1 July 2002.
43 Associated Press, '92-year-old Minnesota man keeps up passion for running', *WEAU News*, 22 July 2017.
44 Interview with the author.
45 Lynn F. Cherkas et al., 'The Association Between Physical Activity in Leisure Time and Leukocyte Telomere Length', *JAMA Internal Medicine*, Vol. 168, No. 2 (2008): 154–8.
46 Xuemei Sui, James N. Laditka, James W. Hardin, Steven N. Blair, 'Estimated functional capacity predicts mortality in older adults', *Journal of the American Geriatrics Society*, Vol. 55, No. 12 (2007): 1940–47.
47 Eliza F. Chakravarty et al., 'Reduced Disability and Mortality Among Aging Runners: A 21-Year Longitudinal Study', *JAMA Internal Medicine*, Vol. 168, No. 15 (2008): 1638–46.
48 Andrew Kingston et al., 'Projections of multi-morbidity in the older population in England to 2035: estimates from the Population Ageing and Care Simulation (PACSim) model', *Age and Ageing*, Vol. 47, No. 3 (2018): 374–80.
49 International Osteoporosis Foundation https://www.iofbonehealth.org/facts-statistics#category-14
50 Interview with the author.
51 Stefania Bandinelli, Yuri Milaneschi, Luigi Ferrucci, 'Chair Stands Test and Survival in the Older Population', *Journal of the American Geriatrics Society*, Vol. 57, No. 11 (2009): 2172–3.
52 Rachel Cooper et al., 'Physical capability in mid-life and survival over 13 years of follow-up: British birth cohort study', *British Medical Journal*, Vol. 348, g2219 (2014).
53 Interview with the author.
54 Official video of how to do the test: https://www.youtube.com/watch?v=MCQ2WA2T2oA
55 Leonardo Barbosa Barreto de Brito et al., 'Ability to sit and rise from the floor as a predictor of all-cause mortality', *European Journal of Preventive Cardiology*, Vol. 21, No. 7 (2014): 892–8.
56 World Health Organization, Dementia Factsheet https://www.who.int/news-room/fact-sheets/detail/dementia
57 Alzheimer's Society, 'How many people have dementia and what is the cost of dementia care?', November 2019 https://www.alzheimers.org.uk/about-us/policy-and-influencing/dementia-scale-impact-numbers

58 Interview with the author.
59 Kirk I. Erickson et al., 'Aerobic Fitness is Associated with Hippocampal Volume in Elderly Humans', *Hippocampus*, Vol. 19, No. 10 (2009): 1030–9.
60 Nicola T. Lautenschlager et al., 'Effect of Physical Activity on Cognitive Function in Older Adults at Risk for Alzheimer Disease: A Randomized Trial', *Journal of the American Medical Association*, Vol. 300, No. 9 (2008): 1027–37.

Chapter 9

1 Joensuu Municipality statistics.
2 Interview with the author.
3 Interview with the author.
4 European Commission, Eurobarometer: Sport and Physical Activity, December 2017 https://ec.europa.eu/commfrontoffice/publicopinion/index.cfm/survey/getsurveydetail/instruments/special/surveyky/2164
5 Interview with the author.
6 Statistics from Pukka Peska et al., 'The North Karelia Project: From North Karelia to National Action', National Institute for Health and Welfare, 2009.
7 Peska et al., 'The North Karelia Project'.
8 Ilkka Vuori, Becky Lankenau, Michael Pratt, 'Physical Activity Policy and Program Development: The Experience in Finland', *Public Health Reports*, Vol. 119, No. 3 (2004): 331–45.
9 Statistics from Joonas Niemi.
10 Interview with the author.
11 Interview with the author.
12 Interview with the author.
13 Health Survey for England 2015: Physical activity in children.
14 Interview with the author.
15 Department for Education's settlement at the Spending Review 2015. For 2019/20, £61.6 billion.
16 Interview with the author.
17 Aubert et al., 'Global Matrix 3.0 Physical Activity Report Card Grades for Children and Youth: Results and Analysis From 49 Countries'.
18 World Health Organization, Slovenia: Physical Activity Fact Sheet https://www.euro.who.int/__data/assets/pdf_file/0007/288124/SLOVENIA-Physical-Activity-Factsheet.pdf
19 Aubert et al., 'Global Matrix 3.0 Physical Activity Report Card Grades for Children and Youth: Results and Analysis From 49 Countries'.
20 Interview with the author.
21 Interview with the author.
22 Interview with the author.

Chapter 10

1 Dr Sabine L. van Elsland, Ryan O'Hare, 'COVID-19: Imperial researchers model likely impact of public health measures', *Imperial College News*, 17 March 2020.
2 Damian Carrington, 'Indoor and outdoor air pollution "claiming at least 40,000 UK lives a year"', *The Guardian*, 22 February 2016.
3 Fiona Harvey, 'Air pollution: UK government loses third court case as plans ruled "unlawful"', *The Guardian*, 21 February 2018.
4 Interview with the author.
5 Interview with the author.
6 Interview with the author.
7 David C. Nieman, 'Coronavirus disease-2019: A tocsin to our aging, unfit, corpulent, and immunodeficient society', *Journal of Sport and Health Science*, Vol. 9, No. 4 (2020): 293–301.
8 Peter Walker, Matthew Taylor, 'Labour to plan green economic rescue from coronavirus crisis', *The Guardian*, 17 May 2020. Interview took place on 15 May.
9 Briefing to political journalists in the daily 'lobby' conference (held via telephone conference call amid coronavirus).
10 Matthew Taylor, 'Large areas of London to be made car-free as lockdown eased', *The Guardian*, 15 May 2020.
11 Interview with the author.
12 Interview with the author.
13 Interview with the author.
14 Interview with the author.
15 Interview with the author.
16 Interview with the author.

ACKNOWLEDGEMENTS

As mentioned several times, I'm not an epidemiologist, or any kind of scientist, so I'm indebted to all the academics and others who talked me through their areas of expertise. I should single out a few for particular thanks. Harvard University's I-Min Lee is probably the world's most renowned expert on – and most prolific researcher into – the perils of inactivity, but found time to speak to me several times, and to answer email queries. Robert Ross and David Dunstan didn't only explain their work, they also tackled my slightly presumptuous personal appeals about, respectively, body fat percentages and how much I sit down.

Richard Mackenzie explained his research on type 2 diabetes, and then very kindly checked the chapter on the physiology of inactivity, suggesting a few tweaks. He also arranged for my battery of physical tests at Roehampton University, expertly conducted by Oana Ancu, one of his research students.

At King's College Hospital, Martin Whyte and Phil Kelly let me follow them on their ward rounds while firing endless questions at them, which they answered with great thought and much wisdom.

I am hugely grateful to all the ministers, officials, experts and everyone else in Finland and Slovenia, who talked me through their countries' efforts to get their populations moving, and to Jan Gehl in Copenhagen. Enormous thanks also to all the politicians and others in the UK who talked to me, not all of whose input is quoted by name.

I researched and wrote this book while working as a journalist during one of the most tumultuous political periods in recent UK history. So thanks to my lovely fellow occupants of room 15 along the parliamentary press gallery corridor, who accepted my occasional disappearances for phone calls with distant academics – *Guardian* colleagues Heather Stewart, Jessica Elgot, Rowena Mason, Rajeev Syal, Kate Proctor, Maria Remle, John Crace and Andrew Sparrow, plus Bloomberg's Rob Hutton. Thanks also to the *Guardian*'s architecture correspondent, Oliver Wainwright, for suggesting people to speak to about movement-friendly cities. I'm also very grateful to Mary Stewart-David, who helped me with a temporary base in which to write.

I'm hugely indebted to my amazing agent, Rachel Mills, who encouraged this book throughout, and had some crucial ideas on how it could be structured.

I am incredibly grateful to Fritha Saunders, my editor at Simon and Schuster, who immediately understood what the book was about, and to Suzanne Baboneau, in charge of adult titles at S&S, who was also immediately enthusiastic and knowledgeable. Many thanks also to Frances Jessop, who led the copyediting process, and her team.

Two very personal thank yous. Firstly to Shelly: the frontline of editing/ideas, who helped to make the book much better than it would have otherwise been and is still the person I still most enjoy talking to. And lastly, thank you to Ralph, who happily went undercover wearing an activity tracker at school, and more generally provided a daily reminder of how vital, intuitive and joyful everyday exertion should be in anyone's life, no matter what your age.

INDEX

index

index

women – *continued*
  modern decline in activity among 19, 22, 24
  obesity and 150, 151, 152, 153, 154, 157, 159, 160, 161, 162–3, 164, 165, 171
  150-minutes of moderate exercise per-week recommendation and 22, 207
  public space and 139–43

sitting and 186
walking and 53–4, 55, 84, 121
World Health Organization (WHO) 22, 47, 52, 98, 151, 152–3, 210
World Obesity Forum 154
Wright, Chris 247–9, 252, 257
Wyllie, Elaine 203–4, 205, 206, 209, 212, 213, 262

Youth Sports Trust 247–9, 251